First-Prize Winner in the American Medical Writers Association Book Awards Competition

"A compelling medical detective story . . . a readable non-technical, and informed account of the history, research, treatment, and sociopolitical concerns surrounding AIDS."

—*Choice*

"Of all the 'non-medical' AIDS books to appear thus far, this volume will be the most readable and interesting for the general public and health professional alike. Fettner's writing style is engaging and direct. Her perspectives are well-informed: her insights are pointed and bold. . . . If you have never read an 'AIDS' book and want a very thorough overview, read this one. If you have read all the AIDS books, this one will complete your understanding."

—Dr. James Deramo, *The New York Native*

"An exemplary chronicle . . . the authors offer a factual and stunning detective story recording the discovery of the condition, the theories as to its etiology, and the unending search for a vaccine or cure."

—*Booklist*

"[A] splendid book, a perfect example of a balanced, intelligent look at a terrible scourge.

Times

The Truth About AIDS

Evolution of an Epidemic

Revised and Updated Edition

Ann Giudici Fettner
AND
William A. Check, Ph.D.

Foreword by Bijan Safai, M.D.

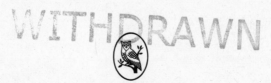

An Owl Book
Holt, Rinehart and Winston | New York

Published by Holt, Rinehart and Winston,
383 Madison Avenue, New York, New York 10017.
Published simultaneously in Canada by Holt, Rinehart
and Winston of Canada, Limited.

Library of Congress Cataloging in Publication Data
Fettner, Ann Giudici.
The truth about AIDS.
"An Owl book."
Bibliography: p.
Includes index.
1. AIDS (Disease)—Popular works. I. Check, William A.
II. Title.
RC607.A26F48 1985   616.97'92   85-17558
ISBN 0-03-005622-5

First published in hardcover by Holt, Rinehart
and Winston in 1984.
First Owl Book Edition—1985
Updated and revised by A.G.F.

Design by Victoria Hartman
Printed in the United States of America
1 3 5 7 9 10 8 6 4 2

ISBN 0-03-005622-5

For my children, their children, and
the memory of Beatrice Ambasa of Marigoli
—A.G.F.

For my wife and children
—W.A.C.

Contents

vii

Acknowledgments

Help comes in many forms. My thanks to Jo Cauthorn, Nancy Cole, Dr. Richard Dijoia, Steve and Belle Fettner, Augustus Goertz, Jim Graham, Joan Granucci-Lesser, Linda Huggins, Larry Medley, Charles Ortlieb, Maurice Rosen, Susan Steinmetz, Dr. and Mrs. David Vastine, Susan and B. Wardlaw, and to my staunch editor, Paul Bresnick.

—*Ann Giudici Fettner*

I would like to thank the researchers, clinicians, and patients who were kind enough to take time to speak with us in the midst of their busy lives. Without them, this would not be the story of AIDS.

I would also like to express my deep appreciation to my wife, Irene, for many helpful discussions and ideas and for doing the work of two during the writing of this book. And to my children for not being too insistent on getting their fair share of attention.

—*William A. Check*

Foreword

For over four years, our society has been faced with a major epidemic. The Acquired Immune Deficiency Syndrome, or AIDS—named for the progressive loss of immune function in its victims—has sickened or killed thousands of people worldwide, and the mortality rate is virtually as high today as it was four years ago. In a world where the great advances in medical science and technology over the past few decades had made physicians confident that the infectious diseases of mankind were both curable and largely under control, AIDS is causing the kind of panic and suffering that we associate with a bygone age.

When the exquisitely complex mechanisms of the immune system are functioning normally, they identify, attack, and kill foreign pathogens. When this system fails, as it does in AIDS, the body is helpless against an awesome array of disease processes. The resulting breakdown in immunologic surveillance leads to a wide spectrum of clinical disorders, including the formerly rare cancer Kaposi's sarcoma and life-threatening opportunistic infections. What causes this dysfunction is apparently a newly identified retroviral family. Even though suspicion falls heavily on the HTLV-III/LAV virus, some researchers question whether this agent alone causes AIDS. We still do not know whether the causative agent is new, recently transformed, or recently discovered.

The group most severely devastated has been male homosexuals. For these men, along with the horror of the disease itself, is the knowledge that their life-style is or could well become the cause of their death. Although the psychosocial impact of this fact has forced many homosexual men to re-evaluate and change their social and sexual behavior, others find such modification difficult if not impossible. The observation that the disease can be transmitted through blood products has caused understandable panic in hemophiliacs and others whose lives depend on transfusions.

The tragedy of AIDS extends beyond its original victims. The epidemic has aroused legitimate concern for their own safety among health-care personnel who work daily with the blood and secretions of AIDS patients. The frustration of clinicians, who have to care for these cases but lack knowledge of the disease's cause and preventive or therapeutic measures, is enormous. The epidemic has also put tremendous pressure on the research community to orient their effort toward finding the cause and a cure. Moreover, even if an effective vaccine were available today, it would be three to five years before one could reduce the number of cases. Thus AIDS is here to stay for some time and will continue to cause tremendous concern in our community.

Fortunately, the response from a wide range of health-science professionals nationwide has been positive and strong, as the present volume attests. The technology, talents, and expertise at work on this crisis are unmatched in the history of medicine and may ultimately bring about a major insight into the problem of AIDS. Cruel as it is, the experiment of nature represented by AIDS offers a remarkable challenge to medical science and may provide us in the end with significant new knowledge.

The history of medicine assures us that, with time and effort, this terrible mystery will, like other biological mysteries, be solved and a cure found. Meanwhile, we must continue to hope and work for that day to come. There is also some cause for optimism in the fact that we are, finally, beginning to see an increase in the number of people who have been exposed but have not developed a fatal form of the disease, suggesting that a subclinical form with recovery is possible and that the epidemic will eventually limit itself and subside.

We are still far from the final answer. But as we continue to progress toward it, an account of events that have led to our present knowledge is of great value. The authors of the present volume have compiled a detailed history of AIDS and have given a realistic picture of its dimensions. Their efforts have produced a valuable book, bringing together in chronological form the medical, social, and psychological events of the AIDS epidemic and the struggles that have been generated by them. Presenting different points of view and perspectives on every facet of AIDS, the authors have succeeded in providing us all with a comprehensive and vital document.

Bijan Safai, M.D.
Chief, Dermatology Service,
Memorial Sloan-Kettering Cancer Center
Associate Professor, Department of Dermatology,
Cornell University Medical School
January 1984

Introduction
Dimensions of a Disease

Two hundred and fifty years ago glycerine was first extracted from natural fats in the form of a colorless, sweet, oily liquid and put to use in medicine, lubrication and the manufacture of explosives. Despite supercooling, reheating, and all the usual methods for inducing crystallization, glycerine remained resolutely liquid and it was assumed that the substance had no solid form. Then, early in this century, something strange happened to a barrel of glycerine in transit between the factory in Vienna and the regular client in London.

Due to an unusual combination of movements which occurred, purely by chance, in the barrel, it crystallized.

The client was probably livid but chemists were delighted and began borrowing bits from the barrel to seed their own samples which rapidly solidified at a temperature of eighteen degrees centigrade. Among the first to do so were two scientists who were interested in thermodynamics who had found that soon after their first crystals arrived in the mail and were used successfully for inducing crystallization in an experiment on one sample of glycerine, all other glycerine in their laboratory began to crystallize spontaneously—despite the fact that some was sealed in air-tight containers.

This is a regular occurrence in organic chemistry. Yesterday something was impossible and today it is easy— partly because of the introduction of a new technique, but also in part because of the existence of a new state of mind.

—Lyall Watson
Lifetide

Another crystallization has occurred, its cause unknown, its origins obscure. In different parts of the world, in diverse populations, an organism has, it seems, spontaneously changed its character. It has transformed so thoroughly that it has become unrecognizable: a microscopic *novum*. And this putative new agent has "crystallized" into a deadly new disease—Acquired Immune Deficiency Syndrome.

AIDS is intriguing to scientists, lethal to those affected, and, precisely because it is new and mysterious, frightening to us all. Through time, every person on earth will be touched in some way by what is revealed in the process of plumbing the depths of the AIDS mystery.

Thus far, the only aspect of AIDS that is clear is its *effect*: it is a disease that destroys the very mechanisms by which the body fights off disease. And this, too, is entirely unique: never before has there been a disease that attacks the immune system itself. AIDS upsets the exquisite and dynamic balance of cells that make up our basic defense against disease. AIDS disrupts the equilibrium maintained between "self" and "other," between safety and danger. AIDS infiltrates and sabotages our center for disease control, and foments chaos—immunological anarchy.

It is thought that an unidentified strand of genetic material in its protein envelope—a virus—has caused this. Instead of seeking out and destroying enemies, the foot soldiers of the body's defense forces—the lymphocytes—in the bloodstreams of those infected by this new pathogen are transmitting nonsensical orders back and forth. The result is biological madness: the bodies that give life to these cells and of which they are an integral part die.

Technology has enabled us to make great strides in treating disease in this century, but new diseases have arisen almost apace with those advances. Just in the past few years, we have seen Legionnaire's disease, Lyme arthritis, Kawasaki and toxic shock syndromes. The parvo virus that was known to cause sickness and death in cats recently has jumped a biological fence to infect dogs, and again to cows.

In Africa, Lassa fever, caused by a virus and carried by bush rats, infects children, who, immune to its effects, carry it home to their families. The mortality is high and Lassa is said to kill as many as 20,000 a year. No cure has been found. One hundred, even fifty years ago we would not have heard of this illness. Had a missionary contracted it, he would have died long before reports of his demise from a "fever" worked their way to the coast.

The question arises: Are we merely noticing such events because we have modern techniques with which to detect and evaluate new diseases, or do technology itself and its effects on our life-styles play their own roles in encouraging the development of diseases?

Travelers return from exotic vacations carrying equally exotic organisms, many of which either have been eliminated from Western society or have never been seen on these shores. Scattered reports of tropical bowel diseases, plague, and dengue fever filter into the Centers for Disease Control in Atlanta, Georgia. As populations become increasingly mobile, as air travel takes us in quantum jumps from one world to another, we are likely to see other illnesses caused by agents long sequestered in remote settings, or simply never before encountered by human beings.

Can a scenario such as this explain the sudden appearance of AIDS? Could it be that affluent, highly mobile, adventurous vacationers picked up some rare organism in their travels and spread it upon their return home? Or is it possible that new immigrants—such as the Haitian "boat people"—brought with them a virus to which they were immune, but which was lethal to certain Americans?

While travel has facilitated the spread of AIDS, researchers agree that it is unlikely that the causative agent has been in hiding. Even in equatorial Africa, where some suspicion of the genesis of AIDS is focused, no previous reports of such an illness are known to physicians long treating these populations. But the "dormant agent" theory is still a possibility; no one can rule it out with certainty.

We do know that AIDS was first seen in homosexual men, and that this group has been the most severely affected by the disease. We also know that: heterosexual intravenous drug users contract the disease; men and women of Haitian nationality appear to be at considerable risk; infants likely get it from infected mothers through the umbilical cord; hemophiliacs are contracting AIDS through their use of pooled blood products; recipients of blood transfusions have gotten AIDS. We also know that women can acquire AIDS through normal heterosexual contact, that some otherwise healthy people are carriers of the pathogen and can pass it to others, and that some people who seem to belong to no risk group at all have come down with AIDS.

Although a retrovirus has been implicated as the causative agent, many scientists think that is only part of the story.

For the general public, the pressing question is: Will AIDS spread geometrically until everyone is at risk? With a latency period of perhaps as long as six to eight years, and with more than 15,000 to date having died from, or currently being ill with AIDS, no one can answer this question. Even the development of a vaccine would do nothing to help those already infected.

Furthermore, identifying the causal agent may be less than half the battle. The viral agent that causes polio had been identified long before a vaccine to prevent the disease was finally produced. Flu viruses have been isolated, and vaccines developed, yet we are still unable to keep ahead of the every-other-year flu epidemics: the viral agent seems to mutate after each outbreak and we are always a step behind. Influenza *annually* kills more people than AIDS has over its history.

Even so, flu is a disease we understand; it is a sickness with which we are familiar, even comfortable. If one gets flu, the likelihood is of recovery. This is not the case with AIDS: when this disease is diagnosed and confirmed, the likelihood is of death—perhaps lingering, sometimes quick.

AIDS strikes at the very heart of health—the immune system. The *symptoms* of AIDS include the disease of which we are most frightened—cancer. Another symptom is an especially virulent type of pneumonia—a disease for which we assume we had adequate medical treatment. And in the wake of AIDS come a host of esoteric agents, organisms that heretofore were seldom or never a threat to humans; now these same agents are deadly.

We are frightened because of these deaths, and because we don't know what is causing them or how to stop them. And our fear and bafflement are compounded by a unique confusion. The fact that a majority of the early victims of AIDS happen to be sexually active homosexual men has created a social atmosphere of phobia and hostility that itself may be thwarting our progress toward a solution of the medical mystery of AIDS.

"The most striking indication of the pathology of our species," said writer Arthur Koestler, "is the contrast between its unique technological achievements and its equally unique incompetence in the conduct of its social affairs." He equates this with Prometheus reaching out for the stars "with an insane grin on his face and a totem-symbol in his hands."

The physical disease of AIDS has spawned another, rapidly spreading epidemic: AIDS Hysteria. Despite the overwhelming medical evidence indicating that the disorder will remain largely confined to the limited populations that make up more than 70 percent of AIDS victims, the many "touches of the unknown" inherent in the epidemic have created panic in the general public and stigmatized those with the disease much as lepers once were singled out.

Charges have been leveled against gay men for "causing" a plague. They are accused of immorality; the disease is seen as God's righteous wrath. Some do echo the words of Anatole France, who said, "I would rather be guilty of an immoral act than of a cruel one"; but undeniably much cruelty has been done to victims of AIDS in the name of morality.

Seldom have the inner workings of scientific research been played out on such a public stage. With reported cases doubling every six months, and victims dying every week— and a potential public health problem of unprecedented proportions—researchers cannot afford to dwell over their microscopes and contemplate hypotheses. The pressure to produce quick results is intense. As quickly as a new idea or finding surfaces it is snapped up, reported, and entered into the new lexicon generated by the new disease. A phalanx of young men and women have been thrust into positions of heavy responsibility and close public scrutiny. It turns out that scientists are like everyone else—replete with bawdy good humor, suspicions, envy, and talent; they are overworked and underfunded, serious and foolish. Nevertheless, they must conduct their research in a politically charged arena, amid charges of neglect and homophobia, as well as wrangle over allocation of research funding.

Many people feel that since they are not at personal risk of contracting the disease, they can afford not to be concerned about the complex of issues surrounding AIDS. But the reality is that anyone who pays taxes or partakes of the health-delivery system of the country has a stake in the epidemic. All of us who are concerned about cancer, about immune-function diseases such as arthritis, or about illness in general must recognize that solving the AIDS mystery can provide a myriad of crucial insights into the very basis of health in man. Finding the key to the AIDS mystery will unlock many secrets of the immunological process itself.

It must also be emphasized that anyone concerned with the rights of minorities or with civil liberty in general must also have a stake in the outcome of the AIDS story, for its scope obviously goes far beyond that of science alone. An estimated 20 million gay men have been forced by the epidemic to reevaluate both their public and private stances and values. This is a constituency of enormous potential for political clout. The entire country and all its citizens are ultimately affected by any such shift made by large numbers of people with rights on their minds. Such changes affect each of our public institutions.

This book seeks to elucidate many aspects of the AIDS epidemic—scientific, political, social, personal, and human.

Inherent in the unfolding of events over the past several years are the dramas of young people dying from a mysterious illness, and the anguish of their families and friends. But also, the processes by which basic and clinical research is conducted and the progress by small steps to large intuitive leaps in epidemiological science are in themselves the stuff of drama. Since the first cases of AIDS were reported, an impressive array of medical researchers from around the world have gradually joined forces, attracted by a love of science, the need to know, compassion for those afflicted, and of course by the carrot of acclaim awaiting the discoverers of the solution to the AIDS puzzle. One researcher, Dr. Susan Zolla-Pazner, calls the sum of all this talent "the most extraordinary research team in history." Many of the scientists who play a part in this book have long been on research tracks to which AIDS is providing incalculable opportunity. Many others are "just doctors"—men and women who care for and about their patients. All have ideas, private judgments, theories, and opinions. AIDS is their story as much as the story of the patients.

Here is a possible scene from the future:

A young medical student picks up a textbook and begins reading about infectious diseases. The student is struck by one in particular. Not only was its first appearance marked by a special preference for limited populations, but it also was of considerable importance to the discovery of that now well-known fact—that most cancers are initiated by viral agents. The disease was also noteworthy because it was in part responsible for an enormous advance in knowledge about what by now has become routine—the successful treatment of neoplasms. The student studies the pathogen that caused the immune-deficiency disease, learns how it was transmitted and prevented, and that it no longer is found in man. Like smallpox and polio, it has been eradicated. The student turns to a more extensive medical history for background, and follows along as researchers get closer and closer to that point in time described by Arthur Koestler as the "ah-reaction"—the discovery, the solution. The student shakes his young head over the confusion of his elders and muses, "It was all so obvious!"

Knowledge has to do with perspective. Standing at any beginning point the future seems to contain a mathematically unthinkable number of possibilities. Looking backward in time, the chain of events leading to a given discovery appears perfectly clear and simple. The dead ends, the wrong guesses, the frustrations and the confusion, all these are obscured, obviated.

The agony of the victims of AIDS will one day be lost in a welter of numbers. Our medical student will no more concern himself over the deaths of AIDS than we do over the deaths of those who succumbed to the Black Death. He may echo the universal laments of those-who-know when they cast backward and think how simple it would have been . . . for surgeons of the eighteenth century to wash their hands, for instance. But that future medical student will certainly use this disease, as others have used the epidemics of other times, as a pool of learning; he will undoubtedly benefit from the truths about AIDS uncovered by the massive medical search described in the following pages.

1

The Opportunist

> Myths grow like crystals according to their own, re-
> current patterns; but there must be a suitable core
> to start their growth.
> —Arthur Koestler, *The Sleepwalkers*

December is a good month for training residents and
interns. Patients have put off elective surgery until after
the holidays and the house staff, with some free time on their
hands for once, is confident enough after six months on duty
to be able to work without the direct supervision of the consultants. It was just before Christmas 1980 when immunologist
Dr. Michael Gottlieb of UCLA's School of Medicine suggested
to his Fellow, Dr. Howard Schanker, that he hunt up a case
that would be good for teaching about the immune system.

"Most Fellows will say, 'Sure, sure,' then go to the library
and read, but Howard went to the wards and found a thirty-
one-year-old man with a diagnosis of some sort of leukemia,"
Gottlieb recalls. "The man had been admitted through the
medical service with candidiasis of the esophagus so bad he

11

could hardly breathe. His throat was blocked by the fluffy white growth."

The man, Arnold, was a successful artist in Los Angeles and he'd never been sick in his life. To the doctors at the Clinical Center he presented a puzzling constellation of symptoms. Candida, or thrush, is a yeast infection of the skin and mucous membranes that is usually seen only in newborn babies whose immune systems are still immature and in older patients whose immune systems have been depressed by medications or by cancers.

"In this age and type of otherwise healthy patient, oral thrush is as rare as hens' teeth," Gottlieb said, "and we kept waiting for some infection or other to become apparent in him." Arnold had leukopenia, an abnormally low white-blood-cell count. He was also anergic (anergia is a lack of response to test substances that should cause minor skin reactions).

"We looked at his T-cells. Fortunately, Dr. John Fahey was doing research here with the latest technology, so he could do this test for us." What Fahey found was that Arnold's T-helper cell population was virtually gone.

In healthy people viral and fungal diseases are held at bay by the T-lymphocytes. Two kinds of these cells, T-helper lymphocytes and T-suppressor lymphocytes, normally are found in a ratio of two to one, respectively. This ratio has been seen to become slightly imbalanced in many conditions, but the techniques for looking at and enumerating specific T-lymphocyte populations have not been available until very recently—which is why Gottlieb was glad Fahey was around. "None of us had ever seen such a profound T-cell depletion. That really caught my eye but I didn't know what to make of it," says Gottlieb.

No firm diagnosis of what was wrong with Arnold was made; but he was treated for the thrush over the ensuing weeks and recovered enough to be released from the hospital. Within days he was readmitted, this time to the Infectious Disease unit with severe pneumonia. His lungs were so inflamed that he was gasping for breath. Despite standard treatment, Arnold remained very ill.

Then, the first of what Gottlieb calls a "series of serendipitous events" occurred. Dr. Robert Wolf, a first-year intern, insisted on an open-lung biopsy, even though this is an invasive technique with substantial risks for a seriously ill patient. "Dr. Wolf recognized that this was an immunocompromised patient and he argued with the consultants for an aggressive approach. He was right. The diagnosis was pneumocystis carinii pneumonia (PCP), a rare and particularly virulent pulmonary disease, and the Infectious Disease people just stood around shaking their heads," Gottlieb said. Their amazement was over the occurrence of this unusual pneumonia in a previously healthy young man.

Although knowing Arnold had PCP aided in treatment (Gottlieb prescribed a drug called TMX), the diagnosis did little to explain what had gone wrong with his immune system. He quickly developed other infections and died.

Shortly afterward, Dr. Joel Weisman, a private physician in the San Fernando Valley, admitted to UCLA a man in his early thirties who had been ill for three months with daily fevers of 104°, weight loss of more than thirty pounds, and swollen lymph glands. As was Arnold, Al was a homosexual.

"Al was a hardworking man who didn't use drugs and didn't seem to be sexually active outside his steady relationship. He was an unlikely candidate for a severe illness," Weisman says. None of the standard tests and examinations Weisman performed on Al revealed a reason for the wasting illness. The doctor had had Al admitted to another hospital and had treated him with steroids for two months with no improvement in his condition. He continued wasting and developed a severe candida infection. Despite consultation with a UCLA physician, no diagnosis could be made and Al continued on a downhill course. In March 1981, Weisman referred him to UCLA, where he was seen by Gottlieb.

"So here we had two gay men both of whom were virtually devoid of T-helper cells," Gottlieb recounts. "While it certainly was enough to get us thinking in the right direction—we considered there might be something special in their lifestyle—well, two cases just doesn't get you there."

Less than two weeks later, a man named Ron was admitted to UCLA, again referred by Weisman. Gottlieb was confronted with case number 3. He was very much like the others, except "Ron was an IV drug user, a real swinger who had been on a self-destructive binge for two years," according to Weisman. For four months his habits had moderated as he became progressively weaker with high afternoon fevers and swollen lymph nodes in his neck.

"Ron was a carbon copy of the first two men," says Gottlieb. His immune function showed the same abnormalities. In addition cytomegalovirus (CMV), a usually harmless virus that is almost ubiquitous in homosexual men, was cultured from his urine, as it had been from the previous two men. "We tested him, treated him, and released him when he improved. Three days later I got a telephone call: 'Doc, I've been coughing for twenty-four hours and I can hardly breathe.' That was the first time I diagnosed PCP over the telephone. I've done it many times since," Gottlieb says ruefully.

It was becoming clear that these three men represented a frightening disease pattern. But what was causing it? Was it confined to homosexuals? Was it something special to Los Angeles and its vicinity? Was it common in the city? "We began to see ourselves as medical detectives and we looked into everything we could think of that might be significant in the life-styles of the men," says Gottlieb.

Two had routinely used "poppers" (the drugs amyl or butyl nitrite, used by many gays to enhance sexual enjoyment) and had been sexually active with large numbers of other men, many of whom were anonymous contacts met in gay bars and bathhouses. All of the men had high levels of various infections or the antibodies that indicate previous exposure to infections. "What we really thought," Gottlieb recounts, "was that because they went to the baths a lot, they had picked up something there."

Gottlieb took a first step toward answering the questions by beginning a detailed article on the three cases for submission to a medical journal. There, colleagues would read of the peculiar mini-epidemic of PCP and CMV infections in gay men. Perhaps it would alert them to similar cases that might be occurring in their hospitals and practices. Perhaps others had seen isolated cases of the same disorder and would contact UCLA with helpful information.

At the same time, Gottlieb called Dr. Wayne X. Shandera, the Epidemic Intelligence Service (EIS) officer at the Los Angeles City Health Department. The EIS officers represent the Centers for Disease Control (CDC), the Public Health Service's arm for the investigation of disease outbreaks. Young epidemiologists such as Shandera are assigned as liaisons between the CDC and the health departments of major population centers. They both assist local officials with investigations and keep the home office in Atlanta apprised of the status of infectious diseases.

Drs. Gottlieb and Shandera had known one another while Fellows at Stanford Medical School. "We had both moved to Los Angeles the previous July and planned to collaborate on some public health problem with immunologic aspects," Gottlieb says. Adds Shandera, "Mike and I had talked a lot about how to foster better cooperation between academia and public health agencies." They had their chance to do so sooner than either had thought, and with implications neither could then imagine.

Asking Shandera if he had recently heard of any unusual diseases in gay men, Gottlieb specified CMV as the organism that had been found in the three cases he had encountered. "No," replied Shandera, "but I'll take a look around." He did not have to look far. Upstairs in the Health Department's laboratory he found an isolate of CMV growing in a culture. The microbe had been recovered from the lung of a man who had died a month before—of pneumocystis.

Shandera drove out to the Santa Monica hospital where the man had died and examined his records: they revealed that this man, too, had been gay. Back in his office, Shandera began telephoning other hospitals and physicians who were likely to see infectious diseases. At Cedars-Sinai, Dr. Irvin Pozalski said he had a "surprising" case of PCP in a formerly healthy gay man.

That made five. It also made it imperative that word be quickly communicated to others treating infectious diseases. The journal article Gottlieb had written had been accepted for publication, but that would be months in the future. Too slow. So they took the fastest available route to alert the medical community to a possible public health problem— publication in the weekly newsletter *Morbidity and Mortality Weekly Report* (*MMWR*). This small publication is issued by the CDC and circulated nationally to those with an interest in infectious illness. Information received by the CDC can be communicated within a week.

"We sat down in Wayne's apartment one afternoon and

wrote the draft of an article for the *MMWR,*" remembers Gottlieb.

Spinning the Network

The manuscript arrived in Atlanta and was circulated to the division for control of sexually transmitted diseases (STD). The striking characteristic of the report was the sexual orientation of the five men.

"That report hit us right between the eyes," says Dr. James Curran, now coordinator of the CDC's AIDS Task Force. "We had just been working with two other diseases that are very common in homosexual men and that are sexually transmitted—hepatitis B and gonorrhea. So our first thought was that the occurrence of pneumocystis pneumonia in homosexual men might involve sexual transmission."

Curran, and his colleague, Dr. Harold Jaffe, were in the midst of a series of seminars being held across the country to inform public health officials on the latest trends in venereal diseases. The week following their reading of the report from Los Angeles, the CDC doctors held an STD seminar in San Diego. They mentioned the *MMWR* article. "We were discussing it with doctors from San Francisco who care for gay men. Bob Bolan said he'd seen a few cases of the same thing," Curran says.

But Dr. Robert Bolan of Presbyterian Medical Center had no explanation for the rash of infections either. As it was shortly to be discovered, the West Coast was not unique.

In New York, a twenty-nine-year-old man had developed a perianal ulcer that would not heal. He went from one doctor to another; the ulcer was treated, he was given antibiotics and ointments, but it kept growing larger. He began to run fevers as high as 104° and his body was withered from uncontrollable diarrhea and weight loss. At one hospital, a colostomy (the rerouting of the colon) was performed to see if feces might be keeping the growing ulcer infected. The colostomy did nothing. He was given experimental drugs, but they affected his nervous system and had to be discontinued. His physicians tried several weeks of treatment with interferon; it did nothing to change his condition. Then he developed pneumonia.

"They asked me to see him," Dr. Frederick Siegal of Mt. Sinai was quoted as saying. "I found his immune system was strangely, severely depressed. When all the hypotheses we knew to make, when all rational treatment was exhausted, we had to stand around and watch him die."

On June 5, 1981, the report of pneumocystis in Los Angeles appeared in the *MMWR*. "They gave the first page to an article entitled 'Dengue Infections in U.S. Travelers to the Caribbean,' " says Gottlieb. "The CDC wasn't struck enough by ours to make it a front-page item." That perception of the emerging illness would rapidly and permanently change as the extent and severity of the epidemic was revealed.

The week after the *MMWR* report appeared, Curran and Jaffe were back in Atlanta discussing the additional information they had gained on the West Coast with other CDC members. These were pulled together into an ad hoc working group to investigate what the scope might be of the new illness. They decided upon one simple technique—phone calls around the country to inquire if others were seeing unusual illnesses in young men with homosexual orientation.

The epidemiologists' calls turned up no other cases of PCP, but they found something equally striking: physicians in two New York medical centers had seen four gay men with severe ulcers around the anus caused by herpes virus infection.

Genital herpes has been much in the news in recent years, with between 200,000 and 500,000 new cases a year. Although painful and psychologically troubling, herpes generally is not in any way a dangerous disease except for the risk from infected mothers to newborn infants.

But the anal herpes virus infections being experienced in New York by the gay men were light-years beyond what had been seen before. Instead of healing in a week or so, they were persisting for months, continually getting larger and more severe. In some of the men, the infections were spreading from the genital area to the brain.

Dr. Jon Gold, of Memorial Sloan-Kettering Cancer Center, saw some of these early patients. "One patient with whom I became involved was a twenty-nine-year-old operating-room nurse. He was a shy man, born in Ecuador, and reticent to talk about sex. But the people who had worked with him in the hospital said he was gay." (This was the same patient Siegal had had to "watch die.")

"We didn't know what to make of it," says Gold. "Then we had a few other patients with similar features—young gay men with uncontrollable ulcers who later developed infections of the central nervous system with an unusual parasite called toxoplasma, or else got PCP—and we realized that we had probably seen the first case of this type in 1979."

There was no question that the New York patients represented other manifestations of the same immune deficiency reported from California. Two had developed PCP, three had signs of active CMV infection, and two had candida growths. Also, the New York men had the same debilitating early symptoms that were coming to be associated with the illness— severe weight loss, fevers, and swollen lymph nodes.

When Gold, Siegal, and other New York doctors published their report in the *New England Journal of Medicine* in December 1981, they described their patients as "part of a nationwide epidemic of immunodeficiency among male homosexuals."

Of the early days of the epidemic, Gottlieb says, "The original observation was made independently many times. There must have been thirty or forty cases of what we now call AIDS seen in 1980 and 1981 by as many as twenty different doctors. In those early months, something began to dawn in all our minds."

What was dawning was an appreciation of the mysterious and unprecedented severity of the illness. In addition to the related infections already mentioned, the men with this baffling disorder of the immune system were also developing other rare and fatal infections:

- In several men, physicians isolated a cousin of tuberculosis, a bacterium called mycobacterium avium-intracellulare. Even local infections by this pathogen are rare. Only fourteen cases of this disease in adults had been reported in the world medical literature before it was discovered to be growing throughout the bodies of the gay men.
- The brains of some of the men were infected with the fungus cryptococcus, or the protozoan toxoplasma, both unusual infections in man.
- As if to underscore the total vulnerability of the immune system in the new disease, several men were found to have infections caused by a parasite called cryptosporidium, a relative of the parasite that causes malaria. So rare is this organism that only six infections by this one-celled creature were known between 1976 and 1981, according to Dr. Pearl Ma,

an expert on crypto at St. Vincent's Hospital in New York. In 1981 and 1982, Dr. Ma found the organism in fourteen gay men.

Multiple infections with such rare pathogens strongly suggested that this was a new disease. When combined with other unusual features, Jim Curran said, evidence for its novelty was "striking." "Many of these patients were seen at major medical centers by department chairmen and other doctors with enormous experience in infectious disease. They were baffled and befuddled. The head of infectious disease at Sloan-Kettering Cancer Center, Donald Armstrong, told me, 'I've been here for twenty years and I've never seen anything like this before.' "

If anyone was unconvinced that the scattered outbreaks reported to CDC represented a new illness, further proof came from Dr. Dennis Juranek, a CDC expert on parasitic disease. When he saw the first *MMWR* report he went immediately to a file to look up "pentamidine." This is a drug with a limited but important use: for many years it was the only medication effective against PCP. Though slowly being supplanted by the drug used by Gottlieb, TMX, pentamidine is still used by many doctors, particularly as a backup if TMX fails.

Because there is such infrequent need for pentamidine, it is an "orphan" drug, not profitable enough for a pharmaceutical company to distribute. The CDC keeps it in supply from the European manufacturer and sends pentamidine to physicians who request it. All the agency requires is that the doctor tell them what ailment the drug is being used to treat.

When Juranek reviewed requests made during the previous several years, he found that although the actual number of requests had not increased, there were peculiar reasons for the requests. The usual form specifies the underlying medical problem. "Some of the time they check the box for cancer. Or the doctor might indicate that the patient is receiving drugs that suppress the immune system, for instance, after a kidney transplant," said Juranek. But he found that many recent forms had neither of these boxes checked. Instead, he says, "they were checking the 'other' box. They didn't know why their patients were getting pneumocystis infections."

Opportunistic Infections

The boxes on the CDC form represented a range of possible reasons for which patients might ordinarily contract PCP— an opportunistic infection (OI). As the term plainly suggests, these are sicknesses that occur only when a pathogen has the *opportunity* to infect. That opportunity comes when the body's defense mechanism—the immune system—is caught off guard.

A number of diseases, and treatments for some diseases, are known to depress the function of the immune system: cancers often do, as well as radiation and chemical treatment for cancers. Antibiotics, steroids taken for severe arthritis, or drugs given to prevent rejection of a transplanted organ can also create situations in which opportunistic infections may occur. In addition, people who have been badly burned and those with severe viral infections, particularly those caused by the herpes-virus family, are at risk for OI's. Most OI's are minor, but they can be deadly serious, depending on many factors underlying the reasons for the "opportunity."

Some OI's are caused by organisms that normally do not cause illness. A multitude of these organisms—bacteria, fungi, protozoa—make their homes on the inner and outer surfaces of our bodies. We live in a state of uneasy truce with these microorganisms: some appear to have protective qualities (though no one is sure of this). Although all are theoretically capable of causing disease, a healthy adult simply should not get opportunistic infections.

But this is precisely what was happening among gay men in 1981. The thrush seen in the new illness, for instance, while frequently seen in a mild form in newborn infants, was an absolute indication to physicians of an underlying disease— one that was depressing the cellular immune system. None of the men were found to have anything that could reasonably account for this depression.

Starting at Ground Zero

Dr. David Durack, of Duke University, an expert on the relationship between infection and the immune system, wrote in December 1981: "Present indications are that we are seeing a truly new syndrome, not explainable simply by failure to diagnose earlier cases. Therefore, we must suspect that some new factor has distorted the host-parasite relationship."

There were tantalizing clues. The victims seemed to be part of the fast-track gay crowd characterized by frequent, often anonymous sexual encounters in bars, discos, and public baths. Many had said they used "poppers" to enhance orgasm. They also had had multiple repeated infections with various bacteria and viruses (most notably, hepatitis; CMV; Epstein-Barr virus, or EBV, which causes infectious mononucleosis; gonorrhea and other venereal diseases; and amebiasis, an infection of the colon). Could these infections, constantly assaulting the immune system, have somehow contributed to its breakdown? Attention focused on the one virtually every victim had—CMV.

But CMV had its problems. Dr. Durack wrote: "It does not explain why this syndrome is apparently new. Homosexuality is at least as old as humanity, and cytomegalovirus is

presumably not a new pathogen. Were the homosexual con-
temporaries of Plato, Michelangelo and Oscar Wilde subject
to the risk of dying from opportunistic infections?"

In the summer of 1981 all that was known was that young,
gay men were dying of various opportunistic infections for no
apparent reason. Something had entered their lives and their
bodies that was allowing mundane organisms to kill them.
What was the factor? The clues were abundant, as in a detective novel littered with leads. But there was nothing solid
to go on; no way to decide what was real, what mere artifact.

The theme that was to run throughout the years ahead
was established: always an encouraging lead to follow, always
the disappointment at the end of a blind alley.

2

A Most Peculiar Cancer

Resemblances are the shadows of differences.
—Vladimir Nabokov, *Pale Fire*

Joyce Wallace has practiced medicine across the street from St. Vincent's Hospital in New York's Greenwich Village ever since she completed her training at that hospital in 1976. A small woman with cat eyes, both humorous and tough, Wallace sees many of the area's gay men and prostitutes as well as the ordinary stream of patients in a general medical practice.

During the last years of the 1970s Wallace saw "a lot of funny cases that looked as if they might be getting Hodgkin's [a cancer of the lymph system]. . . . In 1980, one of my patients, a really nice gay fifty-two-year-old man, was ill for months with a series of strange, shifting pneumonias, swollen lymph nodes, weakness, unwanted weight loss, malaise. I suspected he might be deficient in vitamin B and when we tested him at St. Vincent's he showed an almost complete loss of B_{12} stores. It would take years to lose it from storage in the liver to that extent," Wallace relates.

25

"We treated him, but he got progressively weaker with severe diarrhea so I put him back in the hospital for an endoscopy [an examination of the interior of the upper stomach]. He was loaded with Kaposi's sarcoma lesions.

"In retrospect, we probably missed the diagnosis of at least two other men with the same disorder. But you just don't see this cancer in such young men. And there were a multitude of other symptoms—such a multitude."

Across town, Dr. Dan William had a sick doctor he was trying to help. "I treated him for intestinal parasites, a disease common in gay men, for two months. But he didn't get any better. He also had symptoms not typical of amebiasis: a twenty-pound weight loss, fevers. I had to put him in the hospital. Though he was a doctor, he was phobic about hospitals, so he checked himself out. A month later he called and said he couldn't breathe."

Back in the hospital, an open-lung biopsy revealed that the young physician had PCP. This was incomprehensible to William, as were the other afflictions from which the man suffered: wasting, diarrhea, perianal herpes virus, cryptococcal meningitis (a pneumonia caused by a rare bacteria). For three and a half months he was in the intensive care unit, much of the time on a respirator to help him breathe.

"He was so upset that sometimes he was suicidal," says William. "And the frustrating thing was that we couldn't tell him what was wrong. We just didn't know what was going on."

The patient was almost identical to those being seen in California, except in one respect: before he died, this man "showed a pigment spot on his nose. We did a biopsy. It was Kaposi's sarcoma. I blanched and thought, 'This is no coincidence,' " remembers Dan William.

"A few weeks later, I saw my next Kaposi's sarcoma (KS) patient. Both men were fast-track gay men. I thought if this was a sexually transmitted disease, we were in for real trouble down the road."

Trouble wasn't down the road: it was down the street in Bellevue. And Joyce Wallace was just about to tap into it.

"When Kaposi's was seen in the biopsy specimen, I called Charles Vogle at the National Institutes of Health (NIH) who suggested I contact Franco Muggia, a cancer expert at New York University Clinical Center," Wallace says. It was the right place to call because Wallace's patient was just like those coming to the attention of Dr. Alvin Friedman-Kien, Professor of Dermatology at NYU.

"It was at the end of March 1981 that a young man was referred to me from another doctor in the city," Friedman-Kien recounts. "He'd been diagnosed as possibly having Hodgkin's lymphoma—enlarged spleen and lymph nodes, weight loss, and fevers of undetermined etiology. He'd been operated on to remove part of the spleen and some nodes, but a diagnosis of Hodgkin's couldn't be confirmed.

"While in the hospital the patient had mentioned that he had these funny spots on his legs. The doctors thought they looked like the kind of bruises you get when you play tennis or walk into a chair and, as the patient was rather athletic, they didn't pay any particular attention.

"He was discharged from the hospital and two weeks later noticed that more of the spots were appearing on his chest and abdomen. He went to another internist, one who refers patients to me. This doctor was suspicious and asked me to do a biopsy—he said he'd not seen this kind of rash before. It turned out to be Kaposi's sarcoma."

Kaposi's Sarcoma

In the United States Kaposi's sarcoma is seen only rarely, in fewer than one in one million people. The disease is so rare that when Drs. Curran and Jaffe first heard of it in connection with PCP, they had only a vague idea of what it was. "We had to go back to the dermatology textbooks for that one," Curran says.

What the textbooks told them was that the overwhelming majority of those who contract this cancer of the small blood vessels of the skin are elderly men of Ashkenazi Jewish or Mediterranean Italian background. Few women or young men get KS. The usual course is a slow, chronic one and the brown or purple spots that signal the disease normally are confined to the legs. Treatment generally is successful and few of these older men die from KS.

As Jim Curran was to note later, "Even a twenty-minute look at the literature showed us that KS is associated with immune suppression." For the most part this means patients who have received kidney transplants. In the few decades since kidney transplants have become possible, three dozen or so cases of KS have been experienced by those receiving the organs. To prevent the immune system from attacking the newly installed kidney, drugs that suppress the immune system are given. This allows KS—an "opportunistic cancer"— to develop. Once the drugs are stopped the immune system returns to normal and the KS disappears. The surveillance theory—that the immune system maintains a watch over aberrant cells that may cause cancers—explains this incidence of KS in transplant patients.

The same cancer is a more serious problem in some parts of equatorial Africa, however, where about 10 percent of all cancers are KS. Usually occurring in men in their forties and fifties, KS can behave either as it does in the West or more as we think a cancer does—by invading other organs and causing death. In African children, Kaposi's is particularly deadly. When accompanied by grossly swollen lymph nodes in the neck, it causes death quickly.

Geometric Progression

The first case of KS seen by Friedman-Kien in early spring 1981 was followed within a week by a second. "The same doctor—who, it turns out, had a primarily gay practice—sent me another patient with similar lesions. But they were all over him and of a darker color. I became very suspicious."

Friedman-Kien observed that the first patient was "obviously homosexual" but no questions regarding his life had been asked. After seeing the next patient, who affirmed that he too was gay, Friedman-Kien telephoned the first patient and began asking questions.

"They turned out to have very similar backgrounds," says Friedman-Kien. "Both were in their late thirties, both had been extremely promiscuous—and into a lot of what is called 'kinky' sex. And both men had a multiplicity of sexual partners over an extended period of time as well as using a variety of recreational drugs—cocaine, marijuana, LSD, THC, MDA, and amyl nitrite, a drug I'd never heard of except for treating cardiac conditions.

"Later, as patients started coming in, it turned out that all of them, 100 percent, had been using amyl nitrite. So the immediate reaction was that not only were they promiscuous, but they'd all been exposed to nitrite. These men also had histories of sexually transmitted diseases—gonorrhea, syphilis, and especially amebiasis. A number had been treated for the amebiasis with Flagyl, a drug which at the time was thought possibly to be a carcinogenic agent."

In his years as a professor of dermatology at five institutions, Friedman-Kien had seen perhaps thirty cases of Kaposi's, all in elderly men. The Cancer Registry at New York University showed no cases of KS in patients under the age of fifty at Bellevue Hospital during the nine years previous to 1979. To see such a rare disorder twice in ten days was something he felt must be followed up, so Dr. Friedman-Kien began putting out feelers. Getting a list of doctors with gay practices from the Gay Men's Health Clinic on Manhattan's Lower East Side, he wrote each to inquire if they had had recent experience with patients resembling the ones at NYU.

"Within ten days, I had seen six more cases," he says. At the same time he learned of Dr. Linda Laubenstein's patients at his own institution. "She didn't realize that the men were gay," he says, "but, well, you know, back then you didn't ask people those questions very often—now one does."

Friedman-Kien also learned that a half dozen similar cases had been seen at Memorial Sloan-Kettering, where it had taken the physicians some time to realize that part of the pattern of these patients' similar illnesses was their sexual orientation.

"The KS we recognized," said dermatologist Bijan Safai of Sloan-Kettering, "but it took a while to connect it to their being gay. Looking back on two patients we had in 1979 and another two in 1980, we knew there was something wrong about these KS cases, that they were very different. The men were younger than they should have been, they were not Italian or Jewish—and they died much faster."

Kaposi's was an illness that Safai had picked for special study at the time he set up Sloan-Kettering's Dermatology service in 1974, and his group had had wide experience with the disorder in renal transplant patients.

"We had already been doing immune-function tests on the transplant patients with KS, so when these young men started coming in, we did the same tests on them. We found profound immune depression," Safai says.

"We found out about their sexual orientation when one of our pathologists, Dr. Carlos Urmacher, was having a four-way telephone conversation with other pathologists—one from NYU, one in Florida, and one from Los Angeles. They were talking over the similarity of the unusual illness in these men and someone mentioned that the autopsy report listed his patient as being homosexual. The others agreed—so did theirs. When Dr. Urmacher told me this, I asked our live patients and found they were gay, too."

Meanwhile, Friedman-Kien was pushing ahead with his survey. He called his friend Dr. Roy Leeper, at the Kaiser Health Foundation in Oakland, California, to ask if he had any knowledge of KS in the large gay San Francisco population. Leeper was to attend a meeting of dermatologists the following day and told Friedman-Kien he'd ask. When Friedman-Kien answered his telephone the next evening, he added another patient to the rapidly growing tally. "Leeper said, 'Jim Groundwater at San Francisco General has a case that sounds exactly like what you've got and the man has got some kind of secondary infection that's very serious. They don't know what it is.' " So did Friedman-Kien's patient. It turned out to be pneumocystis.

"Within a week, Roy called again. 'You won't believe this, but now they've got two cases at Stanford.' "

Looking for Help
All doctors study epidemiology in medical school: it is a science in itself, the specialized study of epidemics. Those who go into this area of medicine use distinctive techniques for tracking and uncovering the causes of disease outbreaks. With

forebodings about what the patients with Kaposi's meant, Friedman-Kien knew it was time to involve those in a position to conduct a more thorough investigation.

"I called a fellow I knew named Ron Roberto, who used to work at the CDC and who was currently in Berkeley at the state of California's epidemiology service, and told him what I was seeing. I needed to know who at CDC I should get in touch with. 'What's common among all the patients?' he asked me. I said, 'Amebiasis.' So Ron gave me the names of the people in the parasitology section."

When the chief of the parasitology unit, Dennis Juranek, received Dr. Friedman-Kien's news, he relayed it to other CDC workers. Soon after, Juranek and James Curran went to New York to look at Friedman-Kien's and Laubenstein's patient records. "By that time we had accumulated nineteen cases," says Friedman-Kien. "There were sixteen in New York and three in San Francisco." The CDC investigators were convinced that these cases were truly Kaposi's.

Friedman-Kien's activities clearly galvanized the recognition of the early outline for the nascent epidemic, but as Joyce Wallace remarked, "Trying to decide who saw the first KS is like trying to decide who invented winter." Jumbled together in the emerging medical corps looking into the new disease were university researchers, general practitioners, and scientists from several disciplines. Recollections of those months are described by various participants as "crazy competition," and "so much backbiting"; rumors spread of patients being co-opted. But as Safai was later to ruefully remark, "There were plenty of cases to go around."

Spring rolled into summer and the cases of KS accumulated. Some men contracted PCP and died; amebic colitis killed one man. Friedman-Kien prepared a report on Kaposi's for the *MMWR* and called *New York Times* medical writer Lawrence Altman with the story. Altman's article appeared in the *Times* the weekend of the Fourth of July 1981 with the headline, "Rare Cancer Seen in 41 Homosexuals." Friedman-Kien's *MMWR* report on Kaposi's followed the California article on pneumocystis by only a few weeks.

"I really thought word of what was happening should get out to New York's gay population," Friedman-Kien explained. "Except for men whose friends or lovers were afflicted, few people were concerned." But Larry Kramer, well-known novelist and screenwriter, was horrified. "Just about every active gay man in New York had symptoms x, y, and z that were reported in the article," says Kramer. "I was terrified, so I went to Dr. Friedman-Kien's office on July 29."

In the doctor's waiting room, Kramer saw a friend who would die less than four months later. And, coming from his own appointment, he encountered another friend, who had just been diagnosed as having Kaposi's sarcoma. "He had a year of agony before he died," Kramer said. "That's the horrible thing about all this. For the most part, staying alive is pretty awful."

Dr. Friedman-Kien was able to tell Kramer that he was well, but he also told him what Kramer had already suspected: new cases were coming in "fast and furious." "Whatever is going on, it's only going to get worse," he predicted.

"Tell me what I can do," Kramer asked. The idea of a gay organization to support research and to inform the gay community of the disease was born that afternoon.

Putting It Together

Ten days later, Larry Kramer held a meeting of eighty men in his Fifth Avenue apartment to hear Friedman-Kien describe his experience and fears of the disease. Journalist Nathan Fain recalls the meeting: "Each man swallowed his panic and—if you were there you recall the exact moment—found himself shocked into action. We would raise funds to back Dr. Friedman-Kien's research."

That night almost $7,000 was raised in a room overlooking Washington Square Park among men who already had a stake in the illness—those they cared about were sick, dying, already dead. The $7,000 turned out to be half the total to be raised by the group for the next six months. Says Friedman-Kien of their activities: "Initially they passed the hat around. Larry Kramer told me they set up a booth right where the ferryboat comes into Fire Island. But most people didn't want to hear about it. 'Don't ruin my weekend,' was the attitude." Not until April 1982 was any substantial support from New York's gay community to develop.

Friedman-Kien went to traditional sources for funding but found them dry. "I was politically naïve then," he says. "I thought if you had a serious health problem people would fund you." He was remarkably successful in raising money from other sources, a success not matched by any other researcher in those early years. He obtained an emergency grant from the American Cancer Society for $50,000 and that, with the money from Kramer's group, "helped us keep the initial research going," he says. In addition, Friedman-Kien was able to secure funds from four private foundations for $10,000 each that first year, support that largely continues.

Across the country, in San Francisco, similar action was being taken by dermatologist Marcus Conant. In private practice and a professor at the University of California, San Francisco, Conant had been instrumental in getting news of the first KS in the Bay area to Friedman-Kien.

"I got a call from Roy Leeper, an old friend. He said Alvin Friedman-Kien, who we had both known for years, had called him to say he'd been seeing young homosexual men with Kaposi's and asked him if he knew of any out here. I told Roy we hadn't, but I could try to find out if anyone else had.

"As it happened, I was giving dermatology grand rounds that week and would be speaking to over a hundred dermatologists from all around the area. I was talking about herpes viruses, which are my specialty. One, CMV, had been associated with Kaposi's, so I used that as a lead-in to ask the doctors if they'd seen any KS. Jim Groundwater said he'd seen one case at St. Francis Hospital." Dr. Conant relayed this news to Leeper and it was passed along to New York.

Then Marc Conant began seeing similar cases. "I expected this problem to get bigger. There are lots of gays in San Francisco, and UCSF is right at the edge of the largest concentration of gay men in the United States—the Castro district. I went to our dermatology chairman, Bill Epstein, and said, 'Bill, let's plan.' "

With Dr. Paul Volboerding of San Francisco General as the clinical coordinator, a Kaposi's clinic was set up in June 1981. "It's been running—and busy—ever since," Conant says.

A Difference in Genes

One of the earliest observations made by Dr. Friedman-Kien was that, like the elderly men who got KS, most of the young patients he was seeing were of Jewish or Italian background. "I said to myself, 'We really should look into the genetics of this disease, the HLA typing.' "

Dr. Pablo Rubinstein of the New York Blood Center was recommended as the best person in the city to perform these complex tests. Within a week after receiving blood samples from NYU he called Friedman-Kien with the surprising re-

sults: almost every patient had the same genetic characteristic—the HLA component called DR5.

It has been said that each of us is born with the disease
that will eventually cause our deaths. What this means is that
the genetic pattern inherited from our parents is unique to
each individual. Coded on it are our biological strengths and
weaknesses—as well as whether we will be tall or fair or male
or female.

One part of this genetic inheritance is a group of genes
called the HLA complex—human leukocyte antigens. As well
as being specific to the individual, certain HLA genes are
more common in different racial groups and appear to dispose
certain populations to different diseases; these markers also
can indicate how populations will respond to those diseases.
In individuals, HLA markers can predispose people to specific
diseases. Men who inherit HLA-DR17 are at high risk for
disorders of the lumbar spine such as ankylosing spondilitis,
or "poker spine," which can cause the individual vertebrae
to fuse into a single, inflexible bone.

Friedman-Kien was well aware that Kaposi's sarcoma had
a particular affinity for men of Italian and Jewish parentage—
65 percent of the classic cases of KS have the HLA-DR5
marker. He had written in the *Annals of Internal Medicine*:
"The association between Kaposi's sarcoma and DR5 appears
to be the strongest evidence in humans for the involvement
of the major histocompatibility system with susceptibility to
a particular type of cancer." With no clear-cut clues as to why
the young men were contracting the skin cancer, Friedman-
Kien felt that the HLA-DR5 marker might represent a good
lead. (But, like so many of the other skeins of evidence in the
developing epidemic, this one was tangled. As the disease
became more common, the proportion of KS patients with
HLA-DR5 dropped from 80 percent to 65 percent, then to

43 percent. The importance of this finding was cast further into doubt by studies in San Francisco, in which HLA-DR5 was not elevated among men with KS, but another HLA marker was.)

The genetic markers offered an intriguing clue, but no explanation for the sudden outbreak of the illness. "I said to Rubinstein that the patients were also getting pneumonias and other infections and that their white counts were very low. He suggested that we started looking at their immune function, starting with how their lymphocytes responded to stimulation in the test tube. That response was clearly abnormal. Then we started looking at the T-helper to T-suppressor ratios and found them to be abnormal, too," Friedman-Kien recalls. Michael Gottlieb had reported the same findings.

In early July 1981, less than four months after the first case of Kaposi's was found in New York, patients were coming in at a rate of one or two a week, and there was no question that a medical crisis of unprecedented character was under way.

More immune studies needed to be done, but Dr. Rubinstein was on vacation, so Friedman-Kien turned to Dr. Susan Zolla-Pazner of the Veterans Administration Hospital, who was an expert in the evaluation of T-cells. "We're not supposed to be doing non-VA stuff here," Zolla-Pazner said, according to Friedman-Kien, but she arranged to have two to three tests a week done for him during the month she would be gone on maternity leave.

"She came back and there were eight or ten cases analyzed," Friedman-Kien says. "The results were so impressively abnormal that she got very excited, and jumped on the bandwagon with us."

One of the things that excited Zolla-Pazner was the reversed ratio of T-4 to T-8 cells (see Chapter 3). What this ratio meant in this new patient population was to remain a puzzle. As Gottlieb had remarked, "There are a wide variety of viruses that produce the same thing—Epstein-Barr and cytomegalovirus—but none of this may have to do with it. If someone were to look at your T-4/T-8 ratio when you have a viral infection, it would probably be diminished."

The Viral Assault

But there were many other aspects of the illness that also were unclear. Why were some of the patients getting opportunistic infections while others were first seen with Kaposi's? Part of the explanation might lie in the HLA-DR5 markers, but this would not be the whole explanation. Many investigators focused in on CMV. Bijan Safai was in a unique position to appreciate the association between KS and CMV. "I met Dr. Gaetano Giraldo in the mid-1970s when he was here from Italy and we combined our work. Gaetano had just shown that CMV was involved in Kaposi's. He had isolated the virus from a Kaposi's tumor, had showed that classic Kaposi's patients had high titers (antibody levels), and had demonstrated that biopsy samples from Kaposi's tumors contained CMV genetic material. So, when we started seeing KS in these gay men, we immediately thought of CMV as a contributing factor," Safai said.

And Dr. Lawrence Drew had just published a paper that showed that more than 90 percent of gay men in San Francisco had evidence of CMV infection at some time—and that many had the virus actively growing in their bodies. As Gottlieb put it, "Homosexuals are assaulted by repeated CMV infections. After each one, they can shed the virus for a year or more. Even healthy homosexuals are frequently shedding CMV, and we don't know why."

But nothing precluded the possibility that CMV was merely an opportunistic infection in the immunosuppressed gay men and that the virus was present as a passenger, rather than the causative agent of KS. Also, all of the sick men, on both coasts, had similar histories of multiple viral, bacterial, fungal, and parasitic diseases. Friedman-Kien was confused by "the enormous titers of EBV and CMV in all of these patients." EBV had previously been implicated in cancers, too.

The question brought up by the presence of CMV, EBV, and the other organisms found in the immune-suppressed men was this: Were these agents simply taking advantage of some wide breach in the immune system's surveillance, taking an opportunity? Or was one, or a combination of several, the actual cause of the disease? Each researcher, according to his or her particular area of interest and expertise, had a slightly different point of view.

A seed was already planted that—keeping pace with the growth of the disease soon to be known as "AIDS"—would flower into an illness of its own. To find the cause of the new illness, every aspect of the lives of its victims would have to be scrutinized. Sexual activities that were distasteful to the majority of the public, life-styles that were mysterious and that included multiple, anonymous sexual contacts in public places, drugs, high incidences of sexually transmitted diseases—all these would soon be grist for the media. The usual sympathy for afflicted people would be withheld, "sick" jokes would proliferate. But it all had to be exposed and examined; the cases were snowballing.

At the end of 1981, Arthur Levine of the National Cancer Institute would write in an article in *Cancer Treatment Reports*: "The mortality rate so far has been 40%. However, more than 70% of patients with the earliest diagnosed cases have died, predicting that the ultimate mortality will be staggering."

Also staggering was the realization that cancer, that most dread of all diseases, was simply a *symptom* of an overwhelming illness that was not understood and on which no medical consensus could be reached.

It was clear that KS was only one of several manifestations of the same epidemic of immune dysfunction. The demographics were exactly the same for the patients who got PCP, KS, or lymphomas (cancer of the lymphoid tissue). And, as Dr. William's first patient clearly showed, the same patient could get both KS and OI.

After seeing two of his first five PCP patients go on to develop Kaposi's sarcoma, Dr. Gottlieb was convinced that there was only one epidemic with protean manifestations. "It was just coincidence that it was reported as opportunistic infections on the West Coast and skin cancer in New York," he says. "It happens that it was picked up first in New York by dermatologists and oncologists, and they concentrated on the skin cancer. We focused on the unusual pneumonia and the immune system defects. But it seemed clear to me from the start that it was one epidemic, and that KS was only one of many lethal diseases striking young gay men."

The doctors could agree on the nature and scope of the problem, but they could not agree on a course of action. Friedman-Kien said that part of what was missing was "collaborative efforts that could have gone through had people been more cooperative."

But nothing was cooperating. Each of the cancers and each of the infections that were assaulting the men had a known treatment; but as one sickness was cured, another appeared. The medications that helped one man were ineffectual in an identical case. The disease itself was not the cancers, the opportunistic infections. Those were merely indications of the underlying disorder. Something bizarre had happened to that function of the body on which all health depends—the immune system.

3

A Delicate Balance:
The Immune System

Things fall apart; the center cannot hold;
Mere anarchy is loosed upon the world.
—W. B. Yeats,
"The Second Coming"

Brisk, precise Anthony Fauci is not easily rattled. As a prominent research immunologist at the National Institutes of Health, with a special interest in autoimmune phenomena, Fauci has come across many peculiar manifestations of immune-system malfunction. But Dr. Fauci was indeed rattled when he encountered AIDS.

"When I first read about the California cases in the June 1981 *MMWR*, I thought, 'Fluke! They probably have ingested some bad drugs,' and I just forgot about it. Then the July issue came out: the pneumocystis had been joined by Kaposi's and I thought, 'Oops! This is strange!' Then I started hearing things from my colleagues in New York and, knowing the sexual exposure of gay men, I became vaguely anxious that it might be a new disease—and that it would spread."

When Fauci looked at the immune function of the first

AIDS patient admitted to the NIH Clinical Center in Bethesda, he saw two things he'd never seen before: "The first was that, while opportunistic infections usually affect people with across-the-board immune suppression, this one was very selective. The second was absolutely new to me: certain lymphocytes, the T-4 cells, that should have been there were simply gone, absent."

Fauci's colleague at NIH, Dr. Arthur Levine, amplifies: "None of these individual diseases is new. Most are caused by infectious agents long present in the population and against which most adult Americans have developed resistance. The several diseases designated AIDS are in fact old cohabitors of our bodies.

"In AIDS patients the traditional treatments aren't working because these diseases are the symptoms of a depressed immune system. The patients are going to continue having these 'symptoms' even if you put the Kaposi's sarcoma into remission or clear up the infection. Whatever provoked it in the first place is still there. The appearance of these diseases in often-lethal form is a symptom of the underlying disease—the first epidemic of profoundly depressed immune systems. We work backward from what we see to how things might have gotten that way."

The Immune Defense

The human body is an intricate collection of interrelated systems whose ultimate functions are to protect life. Humans are not endowed with the elaborate camouflage, the great speed or size, or the poison or painful spines of other creatures. Nonetheless, we are equipped with an elaborate and highly efficient defense system.

The first and most obvious element is the twenty-one square feet of skin that make up our largest organ. When the integrity of the skin is lost through a scrape or cut, organisms that live on its surface are allowed to invade. When this occurs, another protective mechanism comes into play—the immune system, headquartered in the white cells of the bloodstream, the staging ground for a cellular army.

A small cut is a trivial skirmish for the immune system, but even that involves millions of cells and a host of chemical events to rid the tissues of the microorganisms that, if unchecked, could kill. And, of course, germs taken in with air or ingested with food also bypass the skin barrier. But by whatever route of entry, all that passes into our bodies is inspected and evaluated by the front-line guardians of health—the white blood cells, which, together with the fluid in which they live, make up the process called the immune system.

The immune function is created by the activity of the several kinds of white cells. Most types of white cells will attack anything recognized by them as "other." But one—the lymphocyte—is special; the body's ultimate defense depends on lymphocytes and their offspring.

The two types of lymphocytes are programmed to lie in wait exclusively for very specific substances. These are the B-cells and the T-cells that form what is known as the two "arms" of the immune system. The B-cell arm produces the antibody proteins which identify invaders and which begin the processes that lead to their destruction. On the surface of each B-cell are perhaps as many as one hundred thousand receptors that are like locks. When the B-cell comes into contact with an antigen—a foreign organism or substance—one of these receptors will fit the antigen's "key." This causes a dramatic change in the B-cell: it attaches itself to the invader and begins to grow. It produces a "memory" cell that is also able to reproduce itself, and these lie in wait for subsequent meetings with the antigen that caused them to come into being. Able then to kick off the production of antibody without delay, these memory cells are the basis of vaccination.

But the antibody that B-cells produce is not effective against viruses or bacteria that are able to get *inside* the cells. T-cells have a special ability to resist infectious agents of this class. In addition, much of the action of B-cells is dependent on the function of T-cells.

There are two types of T-cells: T-helper cells encourage B-cells to produce antibody; T-suppressor cells prevent the other cells from overreacting and help limit their activity. (Cytotoxic or "killer" T-cells are probably a class of T-suppressor cells that react with foreign cells.) Both B- and T-cells are sent into action in the presence of antigens.

When the immune system functions correctly, it is able to do a number of specific things: recognize and remember, regulate itself, destroy what it designates "other." Performance of these essential functions involves a host of complex interactions. Our acquaintance with many of these processes is so recent that even those scientists most expert in this area have difficulty comprehending the exact mechanisms.

"We've never before encountered a primary immune-regulatory illness—one that doesn't need a specific infection or antigen to cause immune changes," says Dr. Susanna Cunningham-Rundles of Memorial Sloan-Kettering. "In AIDS any infection will cause a further imbalance in the immune system. It's like a computer that has been programmed so that any input will result in a distorted picture."

Many illnesses severely affect and are in turn affected by the immune system. When the system is overactive, people become sensitive to many allergens, which results in allergic reactions. At the extreme end of overactivity, autoimmune disease can result. For instance, if the red blood cells become coated with autoantibody, they are recognized and destroyed as "other"; the result is severe anemia.

Many AIDS victims have an autoimmune illness called ideopathic thrombocytopenic purpura (ITP); their bodies make antibodies to platelets in their own blood—and this results in oozing of blood from the tiny capillaries. Other AIDS victims have symptoms of other diseases—including several types of cancers—caused by such *over*active immunity.

"But it's only when both arms of the immune system are compromised that we see secondary cancers," says Arthur Levine. "And one type of cancer seen in AIDS patients, lymphoma of the central nervous system, is not even seen in hereditary immune deficiencies. It occurs only in acquired immune deficiencies, such as immunosuppressed renal transplant patients. So we need to find an etiology for AIDS that results in an extreme disturbance of both B- and T-lymphocytes to explain the complete range of diseases we are seeing in AIDS patients."

Renal transplant recipients are immunologically similar to AIDS patients. They have more than one hundred times the usual rate of tumors, including the two cancers most frequently found in AIDS patients, Kaposi's sarcoma and lymphomas. And in 1983 doctors reported that kidney recipients also experience herpes virus and CMV infections in conjunction with helper-to-suppressor lymphocyte ratios less than 1:1. But in the transplant patients, unlike AIDS patients, the cause of the immunosuppression is known. It is the drugs given to prevent the immune system from rejecting the foreign kidney.

None of this is surprising, since we know that B- and T-cells must function together. Dr. Cunningham-Rundles says, "It is very difficult, if not impossible, to say which is the most important part of the immunodeficiency in AIDS because they are all components of an interlocking system. It's like saying, 'Which of the tires on your car would you most like to have blow out?' It's a meaningless question. You need all the tires to drive."

It was easy to demonstrate loss of both B- and T-cell function in AIDS patients. One of the standard tests for immune-system function is for the doctor to inject a small amount of a substance almost everyone has been exposed to under the skin. (This is how the test for tuberculosis is done.) If the immune system is healthy, within twenty-four hours the site of the injection becomes red, swollen, and irritated.

When AIDS patients were tested in this way with various substances, most were unable to form skin reactions. This inability, called anergy, is a sure sign of impaired cellular immunity (T-cells form "cellular" immunity; B-cells, "humoral" immunity). These were substances to which the patients *had* antibody already from having been exposed to the pathogens at some time. But their T-cells couldn't "remember."

Loss of memory was found to have affected the B-cells as well. "Despite the fact that the B-cells are churning out immunoglobulin [antibody]," Tony Fauci said, "they can't learn to make antibody to a new foreign substance. We injected a group of AIDS patients and a group of healthy volunteers with a substance that humans would not ordinarily be exposed to— the oxygen-carrying pigment from the keyhold limpet [a marine mollusk]. When we tested to see whether the subjects' B-cells had learned to make antibody, we found good antibody production by the volunteers' B-cells. But the AIDS patients couldn't make antibody to it. They hadn't even learned to recognize it."

Derangement of the B-cells probably explains why some AIDS patients make antibodies to normal components of their own bodies, just as patients with autoimmune disease do. For instance, Dr. Simon Karpatkin of NYU has found a number of AIDS patients who make destructive antibodies against platelets, the cell fragments that are essential to blood clotting. These men have serious bleeding problems. Other workers have found that some AIDS patients have antibody to their own lymphocytes.

Most researchers believe that these autoimmune signs are a nonspecific result of the derangement of B-cells. Says Dr. Levine, "The B-cells have escaped regulation. They are no longer under control. The result is that they don't behave the way they're supposed to. The B-cells just sit there and do what they know how to do, pump out immunoglobulin, some of which has antibody activity. In this case you'd expect AIDS to act like an autoimmune disease. This easily explains the platelet destruction, for instance."

Reversed Ratios

Of all the abnormalities of the immune system in AIDS, one has received the lion's share of attention—the "helper-suppressor" or T-cell ratio. These two classes of T-cells are distinguished from one another as each reacts with different antibodies. Several companies make antibodies that react with one or the other T-cell, and one of the first reagent testing kits was identified by numbers: Antibody number 4 reacted with T-helper cells; number 8 reacted with T-suppressor cells. Since these products are widely used, the numbers were picked up by scientists who often refer to the "4:8 ratio."

With so many mixed signals, researchers were hard-pressed to find something by which AIDS could be identified and perhaps quantified. The changes in the 4:8 ratio were quickly seized upon as a possible barometer of the disease. Instead of the usual two helpers to one suppressor, those with AIDS had this ratio in reverse. Also, in many with AIDS, the helper cells were almost completely gone.

This was a new test, and researchers like to find a new use for an available technique. But, more important, the ratio reversal was beyond anything seen before. While some infections cause a passing ratio reversal, in AIDS it seemed irreversible and permanent. Dr. Gottlieb finds this still true. "The degree of immune suppression in AIDS patients still looks unique," he says. "Transient reversals of the helper-to-suppressor ratio occur commonly with infections such as CMV and EBV [Epstein-Barr virus] and even some bacterial pneumonias. We knew that already in 1981, when we saw our first AIDS patients. The important point is that in AIDS patients we observed sustained ablation of a lymphocyte subpopulation for as long as a year or more with opportunistic infections. This observation doesn't appear to be spurious. We've seen no spontaneous reversals of these ratios. If anything we've seen worsening of T-helper lymphocyte numbers with time."

The ratio reversal also appeared to indicate the severity of the disease stage. Dr. Stuart Schlossman of Harvard reported a close correlation between how sick AIDS patients were and how badly reversed were their T-cell ratios. In his tests, healthy monogamous gays had normal ratios (2:1); healthy, sexually active gays' ratios were tilted toward a flat balance; patients with swollen nodes, Kaposi's, or opportunistic infections showed profoundly reversed T-cell ratios.

Scientists don't know how to interpret the ratios nor do they agree on what they may or may not mean. "It [4:8] is just another surrogate marker," says one researcher. Another doctor calls the decreases in the 4:8 ratio an "epiphenomenon." According to Dr. Levine, "There is a range of intensity within this syndrome. Some patients have only a modest dropout of helper cells and some have no helper cells at all left.

As with any disease, even a cold, some people will have it not so bad, and others will have it worse."

Others have speculated that the T-4 cells have been so stimulated by previous and present infections as to be unable to respond anymore. With enough T-cells crippled, even a large quantity of antigen might not be enough to cause a response.

Bijan Safai has said, "No one really knows what the 4:8 ratio reversal means. By itself, probably nothing. But the whole thing shows us how ignorant we are about these very important things."

One thing we don't know is why about 80 percent of healthy gay men have 4:8 ratio reversal to some degree. Does this mean that these men are at risk for AIDS? Or do 4:8 ratios correlate with repeated infections of one kind and another? Might there be a special immune configuration among men with homosexual orientation? At present, there are no answers to these questions, but there is much speculation.

Michael Gottlieb and others have reported a difference in the T-cell ratio conformation in gay men who are healthy and those with any symptoms of AIDS. In the healthy men the T-cell imbalance seems to be caused by an *increase* in T-8 suppressor cells, rather than a loss of T-4 helper cells. In AIDS, T-8 is also increased, but T-4 cells are absent. Common sense hints that the healthy men are successfully holding the immune line against infections. But common sense has been of little use in finding a solution to AIDS.

"One of the real problems is that there is a dearth of information about the general public in terms of helper/suppressor ratios," says Dr. Robert Biggar of the National Cancer Institute. "Helper/suppressor ratio is a brand-new entity. It's been around only since 1980, so there's a whole lot of data tumbling out now relating this to every conceivable disease.

We'll see a lot more of it for the next five years—then the fad will move on. Out of curiosity I had my own typed and at one time it was 1:1, and another time, 1:1.7. The literature says 1:2 is the lower limit of normal, but the actual data on which it's based is very small."

The healthy gay men have ratios much like that of Biggar, who says, "Basically, we can't be sure that a helper cell is a helper cell, or that a suppressor cell is a suppressor cell— because some helpers suppress and some suppressors help." He adds, "And that isn't much help."

So, how useful are T-cell ratio changes for the diagnosis of AIDS?

One of the first researchers to identify the T4:T8 ratio as uniquely depressed in AIDS patients was Dr. Gottlieb. "T4:T8 ratios remain at this time the most helpful single test in the diagnosis of AIDS," he says. "The test is nonspecific in that it is well known to be altered by a variety of infections common in people in groups at risk of AIDS. But in appropriate clinical circumstances, the test can be extremely useful in narrowing a diagnosis. A very low number of T-helper cells that remains depressed over more than two months in an individual with fever, night sweats, and weight loss is very suggestive of evolving AIDS.

"But in healthy members of groups recognized at high risk of AIDS the significance of altered T4:T8 ratios is unclear right now. I think there is no useful purpose in having that test done in healthy people. I've advised against widespread application in healthy individuals of a test with which we have had relatively brief experience."

Dr. Margaret Fischl, the director of the Miami AIDS Task Force, makes the same point more succinctly. "We originally thought that the worse the T-cell abnormality, the worse you'd do. Now we know that's not true. For example, we have seen some patients with PCP who got completely well and others who died in thirty-six hours. They had no difference in immune function. So I think that the helper-to-suppressor ratio is an epiphenomenon."

One gay internist in private practice relates what happens when physicians try to use T-cell ratios to evaluate their own health. "When the first reports appeared that T-cell ratios were reversed in AIDS patients, all the gay docs in San Francisco went out and had their T-cells measured. Then they had to try to figure out what the results meant. I had my own done and they were low. So I worried about what that meant. But I really didn't know. My patients all ask for the test. But I don't draw them anymore. My policy is only to do them in patients who have severe constitutional symptoms.Otherwise it would drive you crazy. It did me."

Mixed Signals

While T-cell imbalance has attracted the most attention, it is significant to note that the environment in which these cells live out their long lives (as long as five years) is also defective. Whether this is merely an indication of sick cells causing other chemical systems to malfunction, or the background of why they are doing so, is an open question. But several chemical substances that are directly involved in T-cell formation and function have been found to be either absent, peculiar, or present in too great quantities.

Interleukin-2. The word "hormone" comes from the Greek word *ormion*, which means "to excite." We usually think of hormones in connection with various sexual functions—androgens, which include testosterone, in males; and estrogens in females. But every body function is affected by hormones. They stimulate a multitude of activities, from overall growth in children to brain function. Many hormones are specific to the immune system.

One of these, interleukin-2 (IL2), is both made by and acts upon lymphocytes. It appears that T-4 cells require interleukin-2 to mature from inactive cells to mature ones.

Dr. Roland Mertelsmann, who has been studying this substance at Sloan-Kettering, says, "At least one reason for the defective growth and function of the lymphocytes in AIDS patients may be the defective IL2 function in them." Mertelsmann found that lymphocytes from AIDS patients made far less IL2 than did those from healthy people. In KS, IL2 production was down by half; in those with OI's, 90 percent of IL2 was gone.

Interferon. Another chemical malfunction of AIDS is found in interferon. Although it was first isolated as a natural antivirus substance, interferon has recently been shown to be a signal for cell growth factor as well. There are probably more than fifty interferons.

Dr. Jan Vilcek of NYU has detected strange interferon activity in the blood of AIDS patients. "Since these patients have multiple viral infections, we expected to see the typical interferons that the lymphocytes produce when virus is present. Instead, in about half the patients we found an unusual form of this type of interferon made by the white blood cells. The interesting thing about this molecule [interferon] is that it is also found in persons with autoimmune diseases, particularly lupus."

Thymosin. A third substance found to behave erratically in AIDS is the immune hormone called thymosin. When prototype lymphocyte cells are released from the bone marrow in which they originate, those destined to be T-lymphocytes must pass through (and be changed by) the thymus gland from which they get their "T" designation. The thymus, a small collection of tissue situated behind the breastbone, actively processes these cells.

Dr. Allan Goldstein, of George Washington University School of Medicine in the District of Columbia, was one of the codiscoverers of thymosin in the 1960s. "I have been interested for the past twenty years in the mechanism by which the thymus controls the immune system," says Goldstein. "We found that the thymus produces a family of hormones, the thymosins. There may be as many as twenty of these related hormones. It is these hormones, secreted by the thymus, that control the maturation of immature cells into mature T-cells."

In late 1980 Dr. Peter Mansell, of M. D. Anderson Hospital in Houston, Texas, sent blood samples from five AIDS patients to Goldstein, asking that they be tested for thymosin levels. Mansell wondered whether the lack of T-cell function in AIDS might be due to deficient levels of the hormone. In particular, he expected low levels of thymosin-alpha-1, the form most important to T-helper maturation.

"Very much to our surprise," Goldstein says, "we found just the opposite—there was more than twice the amount of thymosin-alpha-1 normally seen in blood. We have seen this elevation now in 70 to 80 percent of AIDS patients." Goldstein thinks there are several possible reasons for these high levels. "The rise of thymosin levels may reflect a disturbance in the function of the thymus, or may be a consequence of the defective T-4 cells. Normally, these cells send a signal back to the thymus to stop producing the hormone, but they may no longer be able to do so."

Goldstein contacted the CDC to see what the thymus glands of AIDS patients had been found to be like. To his chagrin, he was told that no one had looked at them because, to quote Goldstein, "they seemed to be under the impression that the thymus had no function after infancy."

Possible Effects of Stress

In a 1981 article in *Science*, Goldstein, with Dr. Robert Rebar of the University of California at San Diego, showed that thymosin directly stimulates an area of the brain to release a hormone that interacts with the immune system. "There is no question," Goldstein says, "that there is a brain connection between the immune system, stress, and some of the other endocrine systems."

For years there has been speculation that the immune system is at least partially under the control of the unconscious mind. Though this whole area of possibility is murky and poorly researched, there are many indications of such a possibility.

Why, for instance, do those recently widowed have a higher than expected incidence of cancer? Also, two recent studies reported in the *Journal of the American Medical Association* (*JAMA*) measured the activity of lymphocytes in men whose wives had died of breast cancer. They disclosed a "significant decline" in the activity of these cells. "Suppression of the immune system may [also] be affected by the neurochemical mechanisms that have been associated with depression and anxiety," reported Dr. Steven Schleifer of Mt. Sinai School of Medicine in New York.

British researchers recently reported in *Lancet* that the immune systems of dental students rose and fell in direct correlation with the amount of stress they were undergoing. The more competitive students tended to show a greater lowering of immunity than did those who were easygoing. What is perceived as "stress" varies from person to person.

It does make sense that, if under hypnosis one can break out with a rash when told he is being touched with an allergic substance such as poison ivy—and is really being touched by a finger or piece of paper—the unconscious must have some directive role that we do not yet fully understand.

Dr. Hal Kooden, a New York psychologist whose patients are primarily gay men, states firmly that all of the men with AIDS he has counseled have a recent history of unresolved, stressful situations prior to the development of the illness.

A Special Immune Configuration?

That 80 percent of healthy homosexual men have immune-cell ratios different from those of the general population has concerned and confused researchers. If all gay men with AIDS were "fast lane," if all had constant reinfection by viral agents, the explanation might be that T-cell ratios were upset by the continual fight against infectious agents. But AIDS patients run a gamut of life-styles; and the gay population is by no means infected across the board.

Allan Goldstein, like many others, has speculated on this. "Though I doubt the gay community is at a point now that they want to hear that homosexuality may be a physiological abnormality, indeed, it may be correctable by treatment. I know of no definitive studies that determine whether this could be so, but some of the literature suggests that changes during fetal development may in part account for this sexual orientation."

Many diseases are sex- and race-specific. Might there be something basically different about the immune systems of many gay men that puts them at special risk for AIDS? Scientists are reaching beyond what facts there are to consider such questions.

For ten years, psychologist Ingeborg Ward of Villanova University has been studying the effects of various kinds of stress on pregnant rats to determine what events have happened to those "in whom the anatomical, chromosomal, and behavioral characteristics of typical males and females are intermingled." Ward has found that stressing the mother rats "reduces the amount of testosterone in the male fetuses' testes," which results in female-type sexual behavior.

Other similar studies used various types of stress and all result in adult male rats which assume female mating positions rather than male. The same stress applied to newborn male rats resulted in no such changes. Do such events also affect humans? It appears possible.

Dr. Norman Geschwind, head of the department of neurology at Harvard School of Medicine, is an expert in the relative sizes of the left and right sides of the brain and their effects on learning. He believes his research shows a possible cause for left-handedness and for dyslexia (inability to read properly) and other learning disorders. As the genetic marker for the regulation of the immune system lies near those that determine other characteristics, Geschwind feels there is a possibility that levels of the male hormone, testosterone, affecting fetal development also may have a role in determining sexual orientation in male fetuses.

Excess testosterone production in some fetuses suppresses development of the thymus gland, which is needed to create normal immunity. Dr. Geschwind writes,

> My own guess for a long time has been that the epidemic of AIDS is the result of a mutation of a virus which has adapted itself to some particular immune configuration. This is probably true of most viruses, so that however devastating the epidemic may be, most individuals will not get the disease—or get it in a mild form—but the

special susceptibles to whom the virus is adapted may have very serious difficulties.

Why are homosexuals susceptible? My own guess is that they do, indeed, have a special immune configuration based on the sex hormone status during pregnancy which probably has parallel effects, i.e., both in altering the sexual orientation and also affecting the immune system.

Enter the Epidemiologists

But in the summer of 1981, a far less esoteric search than that for the immune systems' puzzling disorder had to be conducted. For scientists at the Centers for Disease Control in Atlanta, it meant that while others treated dying men and looked through electron microscopes, they had to "hit the streets." What was the extent of the disease? How many were affected? And, of overriding importance to the epidemiologists, could they identify the vector that was transmitting the mysterious illness?

4

The Zigzag Course

> The progress of science is generally regarded as a
> clean, rational advance along a straight, ascending
> line; in fact it has followed a zigzag course, at times
> almost more bewildering than the evolution of po-
> litical thought.
> —Arthur Koestler, *The Sleepwalkers*

"**T**he same week that the *MMWR* reported the pneumocystis in young gay men," Harold Jaffe recalls,
"we were in San Diego for a venereal disease meeting. I was
talking to some of the physicians who care for gay men, discussing what was in the *MMWR* and how strange it was. Bob
Bolan, a doctor from San Francisco, mentioned that he'd heard
of a couple of Kaposi's sarcoma cases in homosexual men there."

When the CDC group returned to Atlanta, a small group
in the VD section met to discuss what had transpired during
the West Coast meetings, and Jaffe mentioned Bolan's KS
cases. The epidemiologists learned that Friedman-Kien had
telephoned from New York to report Kaposi's there. "We were
convinced by July 1981 that there really was something

very peculiar going on, something that couldn't be explained away as an artifact of reporting. We needed to start talking to patients, to *see* the disease, and also to get an impression of their life-styles. We thought there was something obvious going on that we could easily pick up," Jaffe describes.

"Several patients had already died," says Jim Curran. "We decided that the problem demanded serious action and that long-term studies would be needed, so we set up an official task force." The new group would call itself the KSOI (Kaposi's sarcoma/opportunistic infections) Task Force. The term *AIDS* had not yet been coined.

The initial series of interviews of thirty men in California and New York had the same effect on the doctors that actually being with AIDS patients has had on all who have become involved with them. Harold Jaffe says, "At a distance, I don't think we appreciated how sick they were." But interviews did little to elucidate anything specific that might be causing the illness. "It showed us that the nitrites tended to be used during sexual activity and people with large numbers of sex partners tended to be heavy nitrite users. We could see that we would have to do a formal study to dissect out nitrite use from sexual activity," relates Jaffe.

The Centers for Disease Control
The job of tracking down and defusing disease outbreaks in the United States is the task of the various units of the Centers for Disease Control, headquartered in Atlanta, Georgia. Restructured in 1980 into six separate operational units, the CDC was initially organized to control malaria in war zones during the 1940s.

The driving force behind a new role for the epidemiological unit was Dr. Alexander Langmuir, who foresaw the need for doctors trained in the special tactics of finding causes for outbreaks of illness. The increasing mobility of Americans meant that state and national boundaries would be crossed, and that illnesses of foreign origin were likely to enter this country. State and local health departments in a few places had experts, but there was no national network capable of comprehensive oversight.

Langmuir was able to take advantage of American anxiety during the Cold War years over the possibility of biological warfare. This made it easier to gain federal approval for the establishment of the Epidemic Intelligence Service. EIS personnel are referred to as "officers" since they have a commission in the Public Health Service.

Since its restructuring, the CDC is now comprised of distinct divisions for specific tasks:

- The National Institute for Occupational Safety and Health (NIOSH) is concerned with on-the-job safety and health.
- The Center for Prevention Services (CPS) is responsible for immunization programs, operates quarantine stations, and oversees the incidence of tuberculosis. This unit also deals with sexually transmitted diseases such as gonorrhea and syphilis, and was at the center of the swine-flu fiasco during Gerald Ford's presidency.
- The Center for Health Promotion and Education (CHPE) is responsible for monitoring possible "habit" illnesses such as a link between the Pill and cancer.
- The Center for Environmental Health (CEH) studies diseases related to the environment. This division studies, for example, possible cancer-chemical

connections; the CEH has been involved in the Agent
Orange controversy.

• The Center for Professional Development is involved with the training of in-house personnel to
enhance skills and knowledge of health workers.

• The Center for Infectious Diseases (CID) has
more than a dozen sections, concerned with tracking
communicable illnesses such as Legionnaire's disease and toxic shock syndrome. The CID also monitors diseases such as yellow fever and cholera, flu,
and unexplained fevers, as well as morbidity that
appears in clusters of new populations. It is this unit
that has prime responsibility for the epidemiology
of AIDS.

In the decades since Langmuir's revamping of this government agency, the CDC has traced hepatitis to contaminated cream donuts, food poisoning to undercooked pork
sausage (the classic "church supper" outbreak); intestinal parasites to organisms in raw fish, and a fatal anthrax to house
insulation made with goat hair that harbored the deadly spores.

More recently, the medical detectives have aided in the
epidemiology of deadly Lassa fever in Africa, finding that bush
rats escaping from burned underbrush were passing the viral
agent to children who captured them. The children, though
not ill themselves, passed the virus to their adult family members. No preventive for Lassa fever has been found since the
agent was discovered in the mid-1970s.

In West Virginia and Michigan, CDC officers discovered
that an outbreak of diarrhea in young people was due to a
pathogen that contaminated marijuana stored in chicken coops.

Perhaps the two most notable CDC achievements are
microbiologist Joseph McDade's identification of the organism
that caused the 1976 Legionnaire's pneumonia in Philadel-

phia, and Dr. Katherine Shands's finding that superabsorbent tampons contributed to toxic shock syndrome.

And, in early 1983, CDC personnel were requested by the Israeli government to investigate the outbreak of nonspecific illness in Arab schoolgirls on the West Bank. They don't always find a bug; this illness turned out to be mass hysteria.

Thus, when the agency reacted to the scattered reports of the strange, and seemingly lethal, disorders among gay men, they were following a familiar pattern, one CDC workers had pursued countless times. But at the outset, no one could have guessed that this investigation would be so different from anything they had done before, and would embroil them in complex social and political problems.

From gays afflicted with a frightening new disease, the CDC came under fire for not beginning work soon enough and for not dedicating enough of its resources to the hunt for the mysterious killer. Physicians who directed blood banks challenged the CDC's reports about possible cases from blood transfusions as "premature." Health workers clamored for guidelines to prevent getting the disease from their patients. In the middle of the epidemic the agency was also fighting for its own life as the newly installed Reagan administration began chipping away at the CDC's budgets.

Whereas the mythical swine-flu epidemic in 1976 had put at their disposal more than one hundred million dollars, this real health emergency posed by AIDS was to be paid for in a grudging, piecemeal fashion, and the CDC found itself in an unfamiliar situation: struggling with other federal agencies and academic researchers over money.

The Task Force

Though many people have been associated with the CDC's efforts in the epidemic, two have been most in the public's eye: James Curran, who was appointed coordinator, and his chief assistant, Harold Jaffe. These young men, both in their thirties, have seemed out of place in congregations of usually much older physicians.

Curran—earnest, bright, and harassed—has been their spokesman. In dark suits, white shirts, and rep ties, Curran resembles a recent graduate of a law school on his way to a political career. Given the difficulties Curran has faced during the years he has directed the CDC AIDS Task Force, no one has suggested that he has done less than his best to deal with admittedly touchy situations. "I've never seen him lose his temper," says CDC Director of Public Information Donald Berreth. "In times of epidemics, when people get panicked, they have always looked to the CDC as a voice of sanity. Jim fills that role nicely for us."

Jaffe has a humorous way of describing his participation in bizarre aspects of the investigation and sometimes seems giddy with boredom at the necessity of repeating the same information over and over to new groups.

If these young doctors and the other members of the KSOI task force had premonitions of the tedious and seemingly endless course of the new outbreak, they were not voiced in those early weeks in June 1981. They did, however, recognize that the number of possible causes of the illness "was beyond the scope of any one unit at CDC," as Curran recalls. What was needed was what the agency uniquely could supply: experts in sexually transmitted diseases, and in behavior, cancer, immunology, bacteriology, virology, parasitology, and other specialties.

First Steps

"When we first heard of the outbreak of pneumocystis among gay men in Los Angeles," Curran relates, "we were faced with three obvious questions: Is it occurring elsewhere? Is it new? Is there a quick and dirty answer?"

The answer to the first question—yes; to the second—probably. But to the third—a resounding no. Contaminated amyl nitrite poppers or an organism newly introduced into the bathhouses would have been the hoped-for "quick and dirty" answer. Identify the infective agent, remove it from circulation, and the illness disappears. For a short time it had seemed as if these were possibilities, but with the disease appearing in several locations, and with numerous different brands of nitrites having been used by the sick men, any such hope was quickly dispelled.

"When something new like this turns up you have to find a place to start. It usually turns out that your first ideas are way off the mark," says Curran. So they sent Harold Jaffe out onto the streets.

"I found myself hanging around Spanish Harlem looking for drugs to buy, and sitting at card tables in neighborhoods in which homosexuals live, asking impertinent questions and trying to get a fix on what it was they might be doing or coming into contact with that was making them so ill," Jaffe says. Street interviews like those conducted by Jaffe were one of the gears that would turn the wheels set into motion in Atlanta that summer.

Telephone calls to and reports from physicians in three cities had established that the illness was appearing in several places. But was it new? Wasn't it possible that some facet of new diagnostic technology had resulted in a coincidental reporting fluke and that what appeared to be a new disease was an artifact of this? According to Curran, Juranek's finding that doctors were checking the "other" box in their requests for pentamidine was evidence that the syndrome was novel. Also, experienced physicians were running into severe and repeated infections with opportunistic pathogens most had never before encountered. All of which was intriguing evidence, but none constituted proof.

The task force wondered whether there had been cases of KS in young men that had failed to come to their attention. For that answer they went back to the telephones. They spoke to people at the National Cancer Institute's master registry; they checked with local tumor registries in ten major cities. Their question: "Have you recorded any cases of Kaposi's sarcoma in men under age fifty?" The answer was often, "Yes, but not before 1980."

Continuing with the telephone surveillance, EIS officers stationed in Atlanta and in seven other cities called doctors at major hospitals to inquire if they had seen opportunistic infections or cancers in young men, particularly those with homosexual orientation. The cities were chosen to include some with high gay populations—New York, Los Angeles, Miami, and Atlanta—as well as others with intermediate numbers of gays, such as Rochester and Albany in New York, and Oklahoma City, thought to have an extremely small homosexual community. Less extensive searches were conducted in ten other cities.

"We asked whether they had had any suspicious cases such as the kinds we were seeing," says Curran. "We found none." But the mounting evidence that this was indeed a new disease was too strong to ignore. "At that point we were quite confident that the problems were new and localized," says Curran.

But that begged the grand question: What was causing the new disease? What Curran refers to as "looking for our tampon" (as in toxic shock syndrome) was not going to be a quick or simple process in this case. The answer—or the lack of it—was to involve the CDC in years of frustrating and often discouraging work.

The Rush to Poppers

"At this point our best clue to the cause of the disease was 'poppers,' " Curran recalls. Originally manufactured as a drug to dilate blood vessels of people suffering from angina pectoris, a painful symptom of heart disease, amyl nitrite came into vogue in the 1960s drug culture. When inhaled, the chemical induces a fast, temporary "rush," often accompanied by disorientation, dizziness, and, because the blood vessels of the eyes are also enlarged, momentary "red" vision. Poppers became especially popular among some gay men because the drug also relaxes the sphincter muscle and prolongs orgasm by dilating the blood vessels to increase the flow of blood to organs. The use of amyl nitrite for these nonmedical purposes quickly brought it under control as a prescription item and made it unavailable except to those with access to the medical world.

Almost at once, amyl's first cousin, butyl nitrite, was manufactured as a "room deodorizer" under names such as "Rush," "Locker Room," "Blackjack," and "Bolt." "Amyl is the champagne; butyl, the beer of the nitrite world," says Robert Biggar of the National Cancer Institute, "and butyl can be made by anyone with a basic knowledge of chemistry." Though most who use the substance refer to it as "amyl nitrite," the majority of what is available on the streets is in the form of butyl.

The possibility that poppers might contribute to the immune dysregulation had come from a "fishing expedition" in which Jaffe and others interviewed surviving patients in New York and San Francisco. In unstructured talks with the patients, the epidemiologists searched for anything the men had been exposed to or had done that had the potential of causing the disease. One feature leaped out at them—more than 90 percent of the men had used poppers regularly.

Fueling the suspicion was an early study by Dr. James

Goedert (and other researchers) of the Environmental Epidemiology Branch of the NIH. In studying fifteen healthy gay men and two men with the illness, Goedert found an intriguing association with nitrites. Half of the healthy men were regular users: all had low T-cell ratios analogous to those of the patients, who were also nitrite users. But the study also revealed that two men who claimed never to have used poppers had the same T-cell ratios. While making a tentative judgment that amyl and/or butyl nitrite probably were immunosuppressive, Goedert admitted that the "tangle" of the nitrites and CMV, and perhaps other infections, would have to be straightened out before any conclusions were drawn.

The confusion of the early days of the search for a risk factor was emphasized by Dr. Biggar: "I went to Denmark to find a population that didn't have this disease. But when I got there, I found the gay men indeed had the same illness. And poppers had been used in the past year by 36 percent of men in cities and around 16 percent of those from small towns." (This is low when compared to about 80 percent of American gay use.)

There were other differences between the American and Danish homosexuals: "Hard drugs were denied without exception," says Biggar, "though about 4 percent or 5 percent used cocaine and marijuana." But there was little correlation between poppers and the immune deficiency disease in Denmark.

Other physicians came up with results different from those reported by Goedert. At St. Lukes–Roosevelt Hospital in New York, Michael Grieco and his colleagues did a similar study. Dr. Michael Lange, a member of the team, summarized the results: "We did not find any correlation between the use of nitrites and a change in the ratio of helper lymphocytes to suppressor lymphocytes." His co-worker, Dr. Hardy

Kornfeld, elaborates: "Among the men we studied, about 20 percent had never used nitrites and about 15 percent used nitrites on a regular basis." Their conclusion: There were no significant differences in the T-cell ratios of the men.

The CDC conducted another round of interviews in Atlanta, San Francisco, and New York: several hundred young gay men as well as heterosexual men were asked about the use of poppers. The results were striking: 85 percent of gay men, but only 15 percent of heterosexual men had used poppers.

But the connection between poppers, gay men, and the new syndrome was not as clear as some had hoped it would be. "Among gay men the use of poppers seemed to correlate with the number of sexual partners," said Jaffe. And Biggar had gotten hints of this in Denmark. "Travel is part of the homosexual life-style, to go around and sample the communities in different places. In Denmark, they make most of their trips to the United States—it's their mecca—particularly New York. A lot of guys I talked to said that New York is a much more swinging place than San Francisco," Biggar reported.

More recently, CDC scientists have obtained evidence that nitrites are not immunosuppressive. "We decided that we really ought to look at what nitrites do to the immune system," Jaffe explains. "We didn't think we could justify a study in humans so we wanted to do an animal study. The temptation is just to do some sort of quick and dirty study and dump a couple of rats into a cage and pour some nitrites on them and draw their blood. But our people decided to do it more thoroughly. First they looked at the toxicity to see what a good dosing range would be. Then they did serial immunologic studies on the mice subjecting them to chronic inhalation. Tom Spira in our lab spent quite a bit of time with people in NIOSH doing that work at special NIOSH facilities in Cincinnati and West Virginia. They started in winter of 1981 and finished in summer of 1983."

The September 9, 1983, issue of *MMWR* reported nitrites had found no effect at all on the immune system.

Sorting It Out

With the evidence that poppers might be a surrogate for or at least have a relationship to the frequency of sexual encounters, the picture was complicated far beyond any possibility of Curran's hoped-for quick identification of some single substance or habit having caused the outbreaks of illness. But poppers were used by *so many* gay men that their possible role had to be explored further.

The classic epidemiologic technique for sorting the red herring from the real is the case-control study. To accomplish this, the CDC selected a number of men suffering from the illness—the cases. To complete the study they selected healthy men who in all other ways resembled the sick—the controls. For each patient there were two controls of the same age and race who lived in the same city. Most of the controls came from VD clinics; the others, from private-practice physicians.

Jaffe says of speaking with these first gays included in the study: "I was struck by the level of cooperation, particularly in the controls [the well men]. The cases you can sort of understand. These are seriously ill people, with a mysterious disease and they would want to be very cooperative. But the controls, who had no vested interest at this point, I thought it remarkable how much they would tell you."

The men were asked to go to what Jaffe describes as "a fleabag hotel south of Market Street [in San Francisco] where I wouldn't particularly want to walk around just for fun. They had to ask for someone they'd never heard of, sit in the room with you for an hour and a half answering all sorts of personal questions, and allow you to draw blood. I don't know if I would have done it!'"

The object of the comparison was simple: to determine whether there was anything about the life-styles of the cases that differed significantly from those of the controls. Armed with a twenty-page questionnaire, CDC team members personally interviewed the 180 men in the study group.

Many of the questions asked in the ninety-minute interviews concerned sexual practices and numbers of partners. The answers given by the patients and controls generated numbers with statistically significant differences. Cases had had an average of 61 different sex partners per year: controls, about 27. For the 50 cases, half of their sexual activity had been anonymous sex with other men, usually in the baths. This 50 percent of cases contrasted with 23 percent of the sex contacts of healthy men from VD clinics being anonymous, and only 4 percent of the sex partners of men from private physicians being strangers.

The men in the study who were ill also had been more likely than the controls to have engaged in the practices called "fisting" and "rimming." These acts involve, respectively, inserting the fist into the rectum of another, and mouth contact with a partner's rectum. While substantial numbers of all of the men in the study had participated in these practices— ranging from 60 percent to 80 percent for rimming, and 30 percent to 50 percent for fisting—those who were sick were more likely than the controls to have performed these acts.

Not surprisingly, those with the greatest number of sexual contacts also had a higher rate of venereal disease and more intestinal parasitic diseases. Several previous studies of the sexual practices of homosexual men had linked specific acts with the development of disease.

Several years earlier, Dr. William Darrow, for twenty years a CDC sociologist, and his colleagues had interviewed 4,300 gay men and had concluded that "homosexual men have higher rates of sexually transmitted diseases than heterosexual men and women because gay men tend to have larger numbers of different sexual partners, more often engage in furtive [anonymous] sexual activities, and more frequently have anal intercourse."

And just a year earlier, a study of men with hepatitis A that appeared in the *New England Journal of Medicine (NEJM)* had shown that oral-anal contact was a significant factor in the transmission of this infectious illness.

For many STD's, including syphilis, gonorrhea, genital herpes, and hepatitis, the risk of contracting the illness is strongly tied to a person's lifetime number of sexual contacts. This also holds true for the likelihood of getting intestinal parasites that cause diarrhea; debilitating bouts of this unpleasant illness have long been dubbed as part of the "gay bowel syndrome."

In analyzing the data from the lengthy questionnaire, statisticians found that cases and controls did not differ significantly in their use of poppers. The picture that emerged inclined thinking at CDC toward another proposition—that the use of poppers correlated with a particular life-style, and that life-style involved considerable sexual activity. Poppers were all but abandoned as a major risk factor by the CDC, though there have been charges that insufficient attention has subsequently been paid this chemical as at least a contributing factor to depressing the immune function.

Harold Jaffe interpreted the results of the case-control study in this way: "We have identified a syndrome associated with a life-style practiced by a subgroup of the homosexual population. The most important feature of this life-style appears to be having sex with a large number of anonymous partners." While this conclusion was consistent with the particular study done early in the epidemic, it also prompted several journalists and social commentators to refer to those men who developed the new illness as "promiscuous," a designation that was to offend many and one that possibly has interfered with accurate reporting.

The combination of the terms "promiscuity" and "risk factors" has been misunderstood by a public for which exactness of expression is vague, at best. Says Marcus Conant, "Many bright people think AIDS is due to something the gay community has done. That is not true. The risk factors are there, but unless a new organism comes along that can thrive under these conditions, there will be no new disease. I remember back in the 1920s hyacinths were introduced into the waterways in Florida. The conditions had always been right for proliferation of hyacinths. But until the flower was introduced, well, they just didn't grow."

Other Possibilities

No good scientist will draw a conclusion based on a single study. Being sexually promiscuous, having large lifetime numbers of sex partners, had emerged as a flashing light in the many thousands of figures generated by the CDC questionnaire. It was an important conclusion; one that needed verification.

In New York, Drs. Laubenstein and Friedman-Kien teamed up with epidemiologist Dr. Michael Marmor at NYU to interview 20 of the men who were suffering from KS. From Dr. Dan William's practice, 40 healthy men were matched as controls. The NYU study addressed one possibility that the CDC study had not: could the incidence of amebiasis and its treatment be playing a part in the immune dysfunction?

"We have the equivalent of heterosexual genital herpes in the gay world—amebiasis," says Larry Kramer. "It was the topic of conversation at every dinner party and brunch for years. It's scary, hard to cure; the medicines are unpleasant and hard on the body, as well as being expensive. Many of the young people aren't able to afford going to the doctor and spending hundreds of dollars just to find out if they're carriers, so they just live with it and continue to fuck—and hope for the best." Kramer also has his suspicions: "Something tells me that the amoebas may have something to do with causing this new disease. . . ."

It was an interesting speculation. Amebiasis is caused by an internal parasite that is easily passed by anal intercourse. And over the years the drug used to treat it, metronidazole (Flagyl), has been suspected, though never proved, to be a cancer-causing agent. With that in mind, the New York group questioned the sick men about the incidence of amebiasis and treatment with metronidazole. They had to conclude that, based on the results, "The hypothesis that exposure to metronidazole might be a necessary step in the development of Kaposi's sarcoma does not appear to be tenable," said Marmor.

In epidemiology, a no is almost as welcome as a yes. It is the "maybes" that remain on the books and in the mind. And those in New York could not quite agree that the popper issue was finished. Was it part of the overall high living of these men, simply an artifact of their life-style? Was the use of nitrites triggering some other recreational drug to cause a lethal combination, one that had novel effects?

Both the patients and healthy men in New York reported the use of many recreational drugs: 90 percent of patients and 43 percent of the healthy men used cocaine; 80 percent of patients and 30 percent of controls had used amphetamines; and 55 percent of patients and 20 percent of controls had used phencyclidine, called PCP or "angel dust."

Experience with nitrite was universal in patients and more than half the controls also had used the poppers. At this point there was confusion between amyl and butyl as perhaps being different enough from one another to cause different problems. Later, however, researchers found that "amyl nitrite" was the designation given to poppers regardless of whether or not it was the drug actually used. (It is this kind of "unknown territory" that often has confused "straight" investigators over the years of the epidemic.)

But aside from the statistical difference in the use of poppers, none of the other drugs used by the sick and well men appeared to have any significant bearing on their conditions. Marmor reasoned, "Amyl nitrite may be a surrogate for another factor, such as overall drug use or exposure to a sexually transmitted oncogenic [cancer-causing] virus at present confined to the homosexual community."

Two Theories Emerge

The numbers developed from the New York survey indicated the same high level of sexual activity among patients as had those generated from the CDC case-control study. Half of the New York patients reported having had sex with ten or more different partners during an average month the year prior to becoming ill. This was three times the amount of sex experienced by the controls. One man in the study estimated he had had sex with an average of ninety different partners a month, while another claimed to "go into the baths on Friday and not come out until Monday morning."

Figures from both the NYU and CDC surveys appeared to link large numbers of sexual partners with the disease in general, and Kaposi's in particular. But epidemiology is only a first step in determining the ultimate question to be answered: *How* did increased sexual activity enhance the chance of getting the disease?

Two answers emerged that have remained the basis of the most frequently cited explanations for the disease: the "antigenic overload" theory and the "specific transmissible agent" theory.

Every time a person gets an infection the immune system stages a response. In one who is repeatedly infected with organisms that cause amebiasis, syphilis, gonorrhea, hepatitis, and other diseases, the immune system must constantly be working to prevent serious illness. "Perhaps," Marmor and his co-workers hypothesized, "multiple and repetitive infections may have caused immunosuppression" that has allowed the development of KS and OI.

Dr. Joseph Sonnabend, a physician with a large gay practice in New York, is one who favors this theory. He feels that "multiple factors, rather than a novel virus, probably induce AIDS in male homosexuals. If this hypothesis is correct, then rational bases for prevention and intervention can be designed."

But Michael Gottlieb objects on the grounds that "people in third-world countries, and some in the U.S., are constantly being challenged with antigens by repeated infections through their lives. This has been true for centuries. Yet no failure of the immune system of this dimension has been documented previously, which is a good argument for a new infectious agent as the cause of this new disease."

The alternative theory holds that a specific infectious agent, such as a virus, is responsible for damaging some part of the immune system's function and making those so infected vulnerable to lethal cancers and rare pathogens. "Perhaps the higher rates of sexually transmitted diseases in patients indicate an increased risk of exposure to a virus," speculated the NYU researchers.

In either case, numbers appear to be an important element. If, for example, two men have sex only with one another, the chances of either picking up STD's or a new virus would be very small. As the number of contacts widens, however, the chance of coming into contact with any and all infective agents would increase proportionately to the number of contacts. Common sense would tell one that the greatest risk is incurred by those with the most different contacts.

But while common sense stands us in good stead for daily living, its value in science is minuscule. Flights of fancy and personal opinion may *suggest*—but they do nothing to prove. The surveys, while highly suggestive, did not prove either an overload theory or the presence of a new infective agent. They also did little to substantiate theories circling around old viral agents or to completely eliminate amyl nitrite as playing a role. This early work raised questions that today are still central to the dilemma of the immune-deficiency disease.

Some physicians insisted that, because the disease was so new, there had to be a new agent causing the initial event leading to immune depression in the gay men. But what *was* it? A virus? A combination of several viral agents? Perhaps a bacteria, or a bacteriophage, a kind of virus that infects bacteria? They speculated that whatever agent it might be, it was rare, probably new, and likely transmitted through gay sexual practices. Moreover, it might have an affinity for some cell that made up the immune defense.

There was a wide range of these agents from which to choose, all of which had been found in the blood of the men who were ill. Virus was popular early on; many are known to cause abnormalities in the immune function. Two, cytomegalovirus and Epstein-Barr, are particularly good at this. All of the ill men had antibodies to CMV and 30 percent in the NYU study reported having had EBV-caused mononucleosis—a rate almost four times that of the healthy gay men studied.

Still, most scientists did not believe either of these ubiquitous agents had been the instigator of the disease. Speaking of a possible role for CMV, Goedert said, "Not unless it's been changed so much that it no longer is the same virus." And neither of the two viruses causes an immune paralysis like the one seen in the men—nor one that does not reverse itself over time. And, as Dr. David Durack pointed out, both of these agents have been around for a long time. The immune-system disease was not seen until, at the earliest, 1978.

The general feeling was that there had to be something new—either an agent or a significant life-style change—to account for the illness. And while researchers interested in the immune system began pricking up their ears, epidemiologists at CDC stepped up their travels into a culture of which they knew very little.

The Mores of a Minority

One of the CDC epidemiologists had been quoted as saying, "Sometimes I felt like I was in a Fellini movie—buying drugs, going to bathhouses." But it was this world that had to be understood to put into context the reports of sexual activities that appeared to be the best clue to emerge from the studies.

The studies had shown that gay men who were ill averaged 500 lifetime sexual contacts—some cases reported many times that number. Those who served as controls also had larger numbers of partners (an average of 250) than estimated for active heterosexual men over a lifetime (about 100 on average). That sexual activity represented a way of life to a subset of gay men became apparent early in the investigation.

The *Random House Dictionary* defines *promiscuous* as

"characterized by frequent and indiscriminate changes of one's sexual partners." This seemed to be what was taking place, but Marcus Conant says, "Overt sexuality is a *statement* of many gay men." And Dr. Weisman cited the unacceptability of homosexuality to society, saying, "If gay coupling were an acceptable life-style, I don't think so much energy would go into looking for new sexual partners." Larry Kramer echoes this: "Sex has become the dominant aspect of homosexual relationships." Sex paraphernalia, advertisements, video cassettes, erotic telephone services, manuals, costumes, a whole host of sex-oriented products and services, as well as bookstores, the baths, and the back rooms of bars, have become prominent features of gay and/or heterosexual life.

The societal pressures leading to this sexual preoccupation are discussed in Chapter 12. To epidemiologists tracking the disease, the important questions concerned the relation of sexual activity to the spread of the epidemic. If there were 20 million gay men in America, did it mean that all were at risk for the illness? How many were sexually active enough to perhaps also contract the disease? Since at the time cases were reported only from the East and West coasts, was there something in the life-styles of these men that differed from men in the rest of the country?

Dr. N. Patrick Hennessey, a dermatologist in New York City, provided some insights into the differences in various U.S. cities. "If someone asked me which large city would have the lowest incidence of the disease, I would say Chicago. For one reason, men who are gay go to Chicago—and stay there." Hennessey explains it this way: "I'm from Michigan, so I had a choice of where to move. As a gay man, if I wanted to move to another environment a little more gay, basically, I'm going to choose Chicago, Los Angeles, San Francisco, New York, Boston, Washington or, more recently, Atlanta or Houston.

But those in Boston, Atlanta, Chicago, and Washington stay put. There is a lot of traveling between New York and California, not the other cities." Says one Southern doctor, "The quality of gay life in the South is different from New York or San Francisco. It's more relaxed. Gay men in Southern cities aren't as sexually active."

A Break in the Bottleneck

There were differences in gay life-styles, but no one knew what to make of them. By the end of the summer of 1981, the CDC and other researchers had accumulated an enormous quantity of data. It was an embarrassment of riches; no one knew how to interpret all the information. Nothing conclusively pointed a finger at anything that represented a hard fact—except that more men were becoming ill and dying. Treatments were working poorly or not at all.

Risk factors included a high level of homosexual activity ("too much sex with too many strangers," said one observer), poppers (at least as a contributing factor), and the multiple infections experienced by many gay men. On this was based the tentative theory that multiple infections "wore out" the immune system. Other researchers thought this was absurd.

Some favored the idea of a single, specific agent; others liked a combination of several agents or factors. CMV and EBV attracted the interest of some scientists, not of others.

Though sex seemed to have something to do with the new syndrome, there were no firm suggestions as to what the connection might be. Despite all of the information that was gathered, all ideas were simply speculations, informed guesses.

At this point, through a combination of serendipity and old-fashioned legwork, a connection among some of the first cases was made. As Curran was to report, "Forty of the first 200 cases were linked by sexual contact." This was a proportion too high to be coincidental. It implied strongly that the disease had an infectious origin and that it was spread via person-to-person contact—sexually. The search for a cause suddenly narrowed and focused on an infectious agent.

5

The Clusters

So far the spotlight has always swung to those who
appear to come up with answers. It's salutary to
consider that perhaps in future the prizes should go
to those people who are able to differentiate between
the questions that have answers and those that do
not.

—David Pilbeam, quoted by
Richard Leakey in
The Making of Mankind

The Los Angeles gay rumor mill began to grind as word
of deaths filtered out and were reported in the gay press.
EIS officer David Auerbach, who had worked on the first
case-control study of the earliest AIDS victims, became the
man to call with questions. Many men called out of concern
for their own health, inquiring whether because so-and-so had
gotten sick, and the caller had had sex with him, was he also
going to develop the disease? And what about his friend who
had also had sex with the sick man?

"It was a surprise," Auerbach said, "we hadn't thought
that most of the men would know the names of many of their

contacts. Then I got a call from Dr. Joel Weisman, who had been helping us with the study. He told me about an interesting conversation he'd had with a man who came to him for syphilis treatment. The man, who was gay, had been at a party some time before where there was a lot of sex. It appeared that eight men who subsequently came down with the new disease had been at the party."

"This man's lover was one of the first Kaposi's sarcoma deaths in Los Angeles," Weisman recalls. "He was naming people who had had sex with each other at the party. All of a sudden, I realized that eight of the patients with the new illness were connected."

If this were true, it could provide an important key to understanding how the disease was spread. Auerbach began checking out the lead Weisman had given him. He first talked to Weisman's patient, got the names of the partygoers, and checked the medical records to verify that the men had subsequently come down with the disease. "Some of it turned out to be true, and some not. But there was enough to justify a formal investigation," says Auerbach.

Dr. William Darrow flew out from Atlanta to work with Auerbach on the new lead. Having been involved in the early nitrite and case-control studies, Darrow was a bit surprised at this naming of names. Although the earlier studies had gone into all manner of questions regarding sexual practices and drug use, no one had asked for the names of contacts. "We didn't think we'd get answers to such a question. And we didn't know how to use such information had we gotten it. It seemed like needless prying," explains Darrow.

At that time, there had been 19 cases of the illness diagnosed in the Los Angeles area; several people had already died. Darrow and Auerbach were able to obtain a sexual history for 13 patients, either from the patients themselves or from close companions of those already dead. Hearsay reports were not accepted; the reported contact had to be confirmed either by the sex partner or by a close friend.

The investigators were amazed to find that "9 of the 13 patients had had sexual contact with other men who had, or later developed, Kaposi's sarcoma or pneumocystis," says Auerbach.

Seven of 11 Los Angeles County patients had had sex with at least one other patient in the County. Two patients living in Orange County had had sex with a man who lived elsewhere but traveled frequently to California.

Even this degree of interconnectedness was probably understated. The CDC report on what was first known as "the L.A. cluster" noted that the other four patients may well have had sexual contact with others who were ill: "One patient with KS had an apparently healthy sexual partner in common with two persons with PCP; one patient with KS reported having had sexual contact with two friends of the non-Californian with KS; and two patients had most of their anonymous contacts [over 80 percent] with persons in bathhouses frequented by other persons in Los Angeles with KS or PCP."

Considering that there are between 200,000 and 400,000 gay men in the Los Angeles area, the chance that 7 of 11 patients would have had sex with any one of the other 6 was remote. There had to be a common factor in their connection. Also, that two KS patients in different parts of Orange County would have had sex with the same out-of-state man was even less likely. The linkage of these men made a compelling case for sexual transmission.

From Coast to Coast
The other end of the unraveling thread lay in New York. In June 1981, Linda Laubenstein and Alvin Friedman-Kien were

"close on the trail of the cases she and I had seen," says Friedman-Kien. "One of these men, who had died, had had sex with a man who had KS, and who traveled a lot for a Canadian company. Call him Erik.

"Someone else also knew that Erik had lived in a house on Fire Island where three men had died. So I said, 'We've got to get hold of him.' Linda said she'd tried to reach him but he'd moved. Erik had been diagnosed in Canada and had not yet become a patient of ours.

"Then I was asked by Marc Conant and Bob Bolan to go out to the first meeting of the Physicians for Human Rights in San Francisco. They knew I knew about Kaposi's and had pictures and slides to show. I went out, gave my talk, then sat down to listen to some of the other talks. A doctor came over to me and said, 'I have a date tonight with a Canadian who has Kaposi's sarcoma. Do you think it's okay for me to go to bed with him?'

"I just stared at him, then said, 'Is it a man named Erik?' 'Yes,' he said, 'do you know him? Isn't he a beauty!' I almost fell off my seat. I said, 'Could you do me a favor? Give him my hotel number and tell him to call me. Or, if he can't do that, to contact me in New York in my office.' I went back to the hotel and called Linda and said, 'Linda, I've located our Typhoid Mary.'

"The doctor called me that evening and said he'd canceled his date but that Erik had promised to call me. He did and came to the office."

Erik had been diagnosed with KS in Canada and told by the physician there that there was no treatment. For eight months he had the typical purple spots but had never felt ill and continued his very active sex life. "In the baths, in the dark, no one could see the spots," he told Friedman-Kien. Linda Laubenstein treated him successfully for KS and subsequently for PCP. He is alive at this time but his condition is getting progressively worse.

When Bill Darrow learned that Erik was a patient at NYU, he flew to New York and found Erik eager to cooperate with the epidemiologic investigation. Erik estimated that he had had an average of 250 sexual contacts a year for the past three years, many of whose names and telephone numbers he had kept. Though it was his habit to occasionally throw out the bits of paper with these names and numbers, Erik was able to provide Darrow with a list of 72 men with whom he'd had sex in the three years before becoming ill. Darrow says, "That was about 10 percent of his total number of sexual contacts during that period."

With Erik's consent, Darrow began contacting the men on the list. "We didn't tell them who had given us their name, we just said we were interested in obtaining the names of *their* sex contacts during the last several years. We wanted to see if they would independently give us back the name of our index case [Erik]. They all did.

"In New York City alone, there were four more biopsy-confirmed cases of the illness among his sexual partners. And many others had enlarged lymph nodes and reversal of T-cell ratios. The time that symptoms appeared after sex with the index case fit perfectly with what was later found to be the latency period of this disease.

"He felt terrible about having made other people sick," says Darrow. "He had come down with Kaposi's but no one ever told him it might be infectious. Even at CDC we didn't know then that it was contagious. It is a general dogma that cancer is not transmissible. Of course, we now know that the underlying immune-system deficiency that allows the cancer to grow is most likely transmissible."

By the time the investigation into Erik's sex contacts was

over, the "L.A. cluster" had become the "L.A.–New York cluster." Said Auerbach: "We have now identified about forty cases in ten cities that we can put on a schematic map that are linked by sexual contact. And we can only guess that that's the minimum number of patients with sexual contacts."

The contacts among the men in the cluster could not be a chance phenomenon. Says Harold Jaffe: "Our statistician tells us that the probability of all these contacts among men with the same rare disease occurring by random chance not only approaches zero—it *is* zero. And that's an unusual statement for a statistician."

The mobility of the relatively affluent gay population became an affirmed factor in tracking the spread of the illness. "We found that people in Los Angeles and Orange Counties were having sex with each other and with men in San Francisco, New York City, Vienna, and other places," said Darrow. "If this is due to an infectious agent," Jaffe adds, "that would be an easy way to spread it."

Around this time, Dr. Jon Gold, infectious disease specialist at Memorial Sloan-Kettering in New York, added another piece to the epidemiological puzzle: "We uncovered a mini-cluster of our own. We were seeing a gay man for lymph-node swelling. He told us about a group of men who had shared a house on Fire Island each summer between 1978 and 1981. Nine of them developed Kaposi's sarcoma or an opportunistic infection. When we questioned them, it became clear that at some time all of them had had sex with someone who had AIDS." Erik had visited frequently in this house.

"I think [Erik] is living proof of the single-agent theory," says Dan William. "The cluster strongly implies that the disease is caused by a communicable agent," agrees Auerbach. "It doesn't prove it, but it gives the theory strong support."

If these doctors are correct, a host of puzzling aspects of

AIDS can be explained. As Auerbach puts it, "The infectious nature of the disease is best seen in the context of the case-control study, in which the number of sexual partners was found to be the strongest risk factor for getting the disease. We can assume that few people had the organism at the outset. The more sex a man had, the more he increased his chances of contact with a man who harbored the agent."

The importance of finding and thoroughly investigating the clusters can be seen in the number of mysteries that were clarified:

- A specific agent or combination of agents was likely, as opposed to the use of poppers or one or another sexual practice.
- One did not have to have a lot of sexual contacts to contract the illness, though most had.
- Many men had been exposed to, but had not contracted, the illness.
- A healthy man evidently could carry the agent with which another could become affected.
- Most important, AIDS is probably spread as an infectious disease, very possibly by a virus.

Too Many—Or the Wrong One?

The most enticing clues that had come from the early case-control study done by CDC were thrown into doubt by the cluster findings. The use of amyl nitrites and the excessive numbers of sexual partners had seemed central to contracting the sickness. Nitrites faded as a leading candidate for the causative agent as men who had had no exposure to them became sick. Although some researchers continue to believe nitrites can be an additional risk factor, few scientists believe they play a primary role.

A similar reevaluation of the high number of sexual partners occurred. The conclusion reached by Frederick Siegal reflected the general consensus: "The strong relation between a high number of sexual partners and the risk of getting this disease was a statistical association. It reflected the likelihood of exposure to an infectious agent."

Michael Gottlieb agrees. "From the first I was convinced that you didn't have to go to the baths to get it. You could get AIDS by having sex with just one person, even your steady partner, if he had the disease."

This probability became more pronounced as time passed and the unknown agent infected more people. In mid-1983, Dan William was seeing a change in patients. "The profile is changing," he said. "There isn't as high a proportion of fast-trackers." But if many gay men have cut back on sexual contacts, why has the number of reported AIDS cases continued to mount so rapidly? "This suggests to me that the agent is becoming more prevalent," concludes William.

Bijan Safai reports the same phenomenon. "Not as many of the patients we see now are as highly sexually active as previously. Before, we thought you needed 150 or more sexual contacts to get AIDS; now we know that you can have five or ten partners and get it."

Says Larry Kramer, succinctly, "All it takes is one wrong hit."

Why Gay Men?

Transmission of AIDS is clearly linked to homosexual contact. Dr. Peter Drotman of the CDC's task force thinks the analogy of AIDS with hepatitis B has merit. "Hepatitis B can be transmitted by both homosexual and heterosexual contact, but transmission is more likely with homosexual contact, which is a more efficient way of swapping bodily fluids."

Sperm is one fluid known to carry viral agents, and itself may be immunosuppressive, according to Drs. Gene Shearer and Uri Hurtenbach of the National Cancer Institute. Under normal circumstances there is a permanent barrier between a man's sperm and his body, a blood-testis barrier. The physical and chemical makeup of the female genitalia are adapted to receive this "biological brew"; not so the rectum.

Studies indicating that gay men who play a passive sexual role have lower T-cell ratios than those who take the penetrative role have raised many questions. Michael Marmor, Ph.D., of NYU said, "I strongly suspect that transmission occurs most readily during anal-genital intercourse," and suggested that gay men refrain from this practice or use condoms. Michael Gottlieb and others have speculated that "an agent in the feces of the passive partner may enter his circulation through breaks in the rectal mucosa during anal-genital intercourse."

The breaks in the rectal lining caused by anal intercourse, and especially the practice of "fisting," can also expose underlying blood vessels to infective agents already present or introduced by sperm. "Rectal intercourse, with its propensity to bleeding, is like an intravenous viral challenge," says Dr. Drew in San Francisco.

"Commercialization of gay sex" is cited by Don Francis of CDC as a contributing factor in the recent epidemic. But he emphasizes that the introduction of a new agent is also a necessary contribution to the creation of the new illness. "If it is a virus that has been lurking in the gay population, it hasn't been lurking long," he says. "We certainly saw an increase in hepatitis B, gonorrhea, syphilis, and other sexually transmitted diseases among homosexual men starting in the early '70s. If the AIDS bug had been there, we would have seen it earlier than 1981. I suspect it was recently introduced and got into the baths and that served as an amplification factor."

Dr. Donald Abrams of San Francisco General Hospital points out that the antigenic-overload theory is especially deficient in explaining why AIDS broke out at the time it did. "It doesn't answer the question, 'Why now?' Most of the viruses that infect homosexual men have been around in that population for a long time. And a high level of homosexual activity is not new."

Michael Gottlieb offers a tentative alternative possibility. "The epidemic of AIDS is clearly new, but AIDS may not be a new disease. Maybe there have been sporadic outbreaks of the disease that went undiagnosed. What's new is that it got introduced into a sexually active population with reduced immunity that served as an amplification factor for it."

Whatever the source and nature of the infectious agent, there seems to be a general agreement that the disease arose at this time because of the increase in sexual activity, the widespread practice of certain sexual acts, and, possibly, reduced immunity among gay men.

Healthy Carriers

A situation which Bill Darrow has run into many times is the mostly monogamous relationship in which one man is well and the other is dying. Because of his personal contact with these men to whom he has spoken before, many call him at the CDC to ask for information and to get emotional support. "We ask these people for information, and they've been very helpful. I think we're obligated to give them information back and to help them through the troubles they're having," he says.

Reminiscent of the guilt-laden survivors of the Holocaust, the healthy men call Darrow to ask, "Why him and not me?"

"The lover of a dying man will say, 'I've lived with him for more than five years and we had sex hundreds of times. I am completely well. Why did he get sick and not me?' Essentially, all I can answer is, 'You're lucky.' "

More scientifically, Darrow speculates that "the disease may only be transmissible during the acute phase of the illness. In addition, the sexual partner of the ill person may be resistant to the infectious agent."

Given the studies that indicate that 80 percent of healthy gay men have reversed T-cell ratios, resistance to the disease might seem a negligible factor. But the assumption that this ratio alone represents being at risk for AIDS ignores an important statistic: less than 1 percent of the gay men in this country have developed the illness. Many more than that small number have been exposed. So, though it has not yet been established what confers immunity, the fact remains— only *some* gay men are at risk for the severe immune-deficiency consequences of AIDS.

The important realization that AIDS could be passed by minimal sexual contacts took some of the onus off those essentially monogamous men who developed the illness. Many had been labeled liars during the time that promiscuity had seemed a prerequisite for contracting AIDS. Also, it began to be apparent that not all who were exposed would become ill, and that some men who knew they had been exposed, though they might have unusual, minor symptoms, would not necessarily progress to the deadly stage of the immune deficiency.

The period of latency, the lag time between exposure and illness, had been expanded by the CDC task force's investigation. What had at first appeared to be an incubation time of perhaps months stretched to two or more years.

All indications pointed to a specific, unknown agent.

Though there are many microorganisms capable of causing infection, none does it with quite the ingenuity of virus.

The Search for Virus "X"

"We live in a dancing matrix of viruses; they dart, rather like bees from organism to organism, from plant to insect to mammal to me and back again, and into the sea, tugging along pieces of this genome, strings of genes from that, transplanting grafts of DNA, passing around heredity as though at a party."

Thus Dr. Lewis Thomas describes viruses, which we are accustomed to thinking about in negative terms. Clearly, a virus is much more than a "bug that causes flu." It is an elegant organism, a stripped-down biological package that carries nothing but the essentials: a strand of genetic information— either ribonucleic acid (RNA) or deoxyribonucleic acid (DNA)— surrounded and protected by a thin shell of protein. Models of efficiency, viruses drift aimlessly until they contact a living organism. Once inside a cell, they use that cell's energy and machinery to replicate.

We are in constant contact with viruses. Most affect us not at all; some cause a herpes cold sore, a wart, measles, mumps, rabies, hepatitis, gastroenteritis, rubella, polio, or the ubiquitous "cold." Of the several hundred viruses that affect humans (animals have their own, though we pass several among the species), most cause no apparent illness. This is fortunate, as we are remarkably unsuccessful in treating viral infections.

Antibiotics are useless against viruses and only in the recent past have new classes of chemicals such as interferon and amautadine been developed to fight viral infections. Vaccines have been developed against some viral diseases, notably smallpox and measles, and work on other preventives goes on.

Viruses have all the properties thought necessary to explain what is known of the disease called AIDS. Some viruses are passed sexually, such as the one that causes hepatitis. They can also cause the kind of slow malaise and constant low-grade fevers with swollen lymph nodes, as in mononucleosis. And a virus called the human T-cell leukemia virus (HTLV) has recently been shown to cause cancer in humans.

But no known virus has ever before attacked specific cells of the immune system, which has led some researchers to speculate that the AIDS virus is really new. Others feel it is most likely a known virus that is for some reason behaving in a novel way.

Given all these equivocal bits of evidence, one can appreciate the frustration of researchers on the trail of a viral agent that could be shown to cause AIDS.

In most infections, the presence of virus can at least be narrowed down by ascertaining what antibodies are active in the blood. The virus enters, and the immune system responds, leaving telltale traces. But, as Dr. Anthony Fauci had said, "AIDS patients seem to be making antibodies to everything for which each is genetically programmed."

At a meeting organized by the National Institutes of Health in spring 1983, men and women who specialize in different categories of viruses were brought together in the hope that an exchange of ideas and information would steer research in a fruitful direction. These researchers would present the pros and cons of "their" viral agent in relationship to AIDS. Some participants were working directly with patients with the immune-deficiency disease, others had had little exposure to the new disease. And, by this time, there had been many theories propounded by doctors to whom AIDS had become an everyday reality.

A virus that is found in most of the adult population has long attracted attention. Cytomegalovirus had been seen in virtually all patients with AIDS, and it had certain properties that were suspicious.

From the first, Dr. Lawrence Drew of San Francisco has been a major proponent of CMV as the AIDS virus. He has been quoted as saying, "If it [CMV] isn't the culprit, it's at least driving the getaway car." His reasons: CMV is endemic in the homosexual population; it is sexually transmitted; it can cause transient changes in the ratio of T-helper to T-suppressor cells; and many patients with AIDS have active CMV infections, some causing death.

But other researchers disagree. Arthur Levine states: "CMV is not what's causing this epidemic. Most people have antibodies against CMV, it's a ubiquitous virus and particularly rife among homosexuals because they have a large amount of reinfection with it. They get this syndrome [AIDS] and it's reactivated even further and they become even more immunodepressed. But it's not the prime mover."

Michael Gottlieb thinks that for such a familiar virus suddenly to start causing a new disease, "it would have had to have changed dramatically." To test this, he sent isolates of CMV from several patients to Dr. Eng Huang, a CMV expert at the University of North Carolina. The results: "No single strain could be implicated. The strains that infected the AIDS patients were the same ones seen in other populations. We found no killer strain of CMV," reported the UNC researchers.

With most virologists unsatisfied with any of the obvious candidates, the NIH meeting was held to interest others with wider experience in the more esoteric viruses. Thirteen different families of viruses were discussed over the two days of the meeting. The tone was best set by William Summers of Yale, who paraphrased Will Rogers: "It ain't what we do know is hurtin' us. It's probably that what we do know— ain't so."

Dr. Usha Mathur of Beth Israel Hospital in New York has been treating AIDS patients almost from the beginning. So it was hard for her to imagine that the virologists were not aware of the potentially infectious nature of the disease. "By their questions," she said, "it was obvious that most of them didn't know anything about AIDS." But the point of the meeting was to get fresh minds considering what had by spring 1983 become almost obsessive to those dealing with patients. And the time had come to alert the entire virology community to the threat AIDS was posing.

The large, comfortable meeting chamber in Bethesda was often in darkness as the audience of scientists viewed slides of damaged tissues, the smudged tracks made by genes, the vicious herpes ulcers, and even a cartoon of a friendly dog to illustrate the talk of Cornell veterinarian L. E. Carmichael.

Dr. Kenneth Takamoto of NIH reported that antibodies to the papovavirus recently shown to cause green monkey fever were found in 27 percent of the population and that gay men with AIDS had "extremely high titers [amounts]" of it. Dr. James Rose of the same institution spoke about a parvo-like virus that causes fevers in healthy people and crises in those with aplastic anemia. Parvo is an animal virus. Had something jumped the species fence?

Dr. Robert Purcell of the NIH described the Delta particle of hepatitis virus that causes disease only when combined with the complete hepatitis-B virus. And scientists were reminded of the discovery of the Rous sarcoma virus, discovered in 1910, which causes cancer in chickens. It took until 1964 to find that without an auxiliary virus, the Rous couldn't "open" the cell wall to do its destructive work.

Dr. Joseph Pagano from North Carolina discussed the suspected linkage between EBV and various cancers and speculated that "if they live long enough, AIDS patients well may develop cancer of the naso-pharynx."

The Prime Suspect

A center of attention at both the NIH meeting and an earlier one at New York University was a subsequently crestfallen young doctor from the National Cancer Institute, Robert Gelman. He had been working with Dr. Robert Gallo, who received the prestigious Lasker award for his identification of the virus, HTLV, that causes human T-cell leukemia.

At the New York meeting, Gelman had presented "hints" of papers to be published in *Science* magazine on the possible relationship between HTLV and AIDS. Refusing to answer detailed questions then, the young man was booed by the audience, made up largely of physicians. Again at the NIH meeting Gelman refused to give details of the work, citing forthcoming publication and peer review. The moderator of the two-day workshop, Dr. Robert Chanock of the NIH, criticized both Gelman and Gallo, saying, "You don't do that with other professionals."

The subject of the secrecy and acrimony was HTLV, a "retrovirus" that has been shown to infect T-lymphocytes. (Unlike other viruses, which contain DNA, retrovirus contains RNA.) When the May 20, 1983, issue of *Science* appeared, four separate studies reported different kinds of evidence for the presence of the virus in AIDS patients. A collaboration between Harvard University and the CDC revealed that 25 percent of 75 AIDS patients studied had antibodies to HTLV in their blood.

Drs. Gallo and Gelman and their co-workers had found part of the HTLV genetic material in the lymphocytes of 2 of 33 AIDS patients. And, working with a group of New York investigators, they isolated the HTLV itself from one patient. The fourth paper, from France, reported isolating a similar virus in a young gay man who had lymphadenopathy but no other symptoms of AIDS.

In the healthy general population, antibodies to HTLV have been found in fewer than 5 percent of people tested.

If HTLV has any relationship to AIDS, its absence in the majority of patients could be accounted for by Gallo and Gelman's observations. "In AIDS patients, lymphocytes containing HTLV gradually disappear," says Gallo. "We found evidence of infection with HTLV in some patients' lymphocytes, then three months later we couldn't find it in those same patients. This is the opposite of what HTLV does when it causes leukemia. Because of this difference, it is a conceptual challenge to explain how HTLV might be causing AIDS. I don't know what the hell is going on."

Allan Goldstein of George Washington University likes HTLV as a candidate based on the elevated levels of thymosin found in AIDS patients. A comparable virus that causes leukemia in cats causes the thymus to atrophy and lose its function, which is what Goldstein believes happens in AIDS.

HTLV has attracted many supporters as a leading candidate, but there is conflicting evidence that points both toward and away from this virus's being the causative agent for AIDS.

HTLV is passed by intimate contact in areas such as Japan and the Caribbean, where the leukemia it causes is endemic. But to date, no cases of AIDS have been seen in the Orient— though there have been a number in the Caribbean. (Dr. Guy Blaudin de The of France reports that between 7 and 12 percent of healthy blood donors in Martinique have antibodies against HTLV. None have developed AIDS.) Susan Zolla-Pazner, who collaborated with Gallo in the isolation of the virus in the one patient, says, "The patient from whom the virus was isolated died of a lymphoma. This lymphoma arose after the HTLV was isolated." Because lymphomas are most often B-cell cancers, Zolla-Pazner thinks, "HTLV, which is a T-cell virus, is not the cause of AIDS, but may be just another opportunistic infection."

And although Michael Gottlieb thinks HTLV in some form represents "the most probable agent," he also says: "It would have to be a variant because the forms of HTLV that we know cause accelerated growth of T-lymphocytes, whereas AIDS patients show loss of those cells." He also speculated that, "If you were measuring antibody response to the right virus, you might see evidence in 100 percent of patients."

But Dr. Margaret Fischl of Miami sounds a note of caution in the interpretation of antibodies found in the blood of AIDS patients. "If you do find antibody [to HTLV], you have to ask if that means that the virus is the cause of the disease or a consequence of the immune dysregulation that is part of the disease process." Many researchers express concern that HTLV—despite its known activity being no different from that of the AIDS agent—is receiving an inappropriate share of time and attention by several agencies. The French variant of HTLV appears a more promising virus, according to immunologist Roger Enlow and others.

Although the NIH meeting did not uncover an AIDS virus, it did serve to alert the virology community to the need for their participation in the search. Dr. Usha Mathur said, "Perhaps it stimulated them to think about ways to search for the infectious agent."

A Recurrent Concern

It is often hard to understand why a scientific community that is capable of sending back pictures from the far side of distant planets is unable to find a disease-marker in a sample of blood known to be infected with that disease. But the planet is out there, visible; all it takes is a means to reach it. Dr. Don Francis of the CDC says, "The AIDS agent is not a standard flu or herpes virus that grows easily. Look at hepatitis A. We never have got that virus to grow. And non-A, non-B hepatitis; we've been working for almost six years with a batch of Factor VIII [a blood product; see Chapter 7] that we *know* is infected and we haven't seen anything yet.

"We have no animal model. We can't just take human livers from patients and chop them up and put them through fancy fractionation. This is a virus that destroys lymphocytes. If the target cells get fewer and fewer as the disease goes on, it becomes harder to isolate the virus."

Francis and his co-workers have inoculated several animal species with samples of tissue from AIDS patients, but after several years none show any signs of the disease. Hope for an animal model may lie in the two monkey colonies in which many animals have died in the past several years from a disease that is both new and appears to be almost identical to AIDS. Researchers have been able to infect healthy monkeys with SAIDS (Simian AIDS) with injections of blood from those with the illness. Attempts are underway at several NIH centers to create the disease in Rhesus monkeys with fluids from human AIDS patients.

(Two articles in *Science* magazine [in January and February 1984] report the infection of healthy Rhesus monkeys with blood from those with SAIDS. In one colony, monkeys sickened and died within ten weeks. In the other, researchers reported finding "a type D retrovirus" resembling HTLV in the infected monkeys. Animal data from SAIDS cannot be directly translated to humans, and attempts to infect animals with human AIDS blood are still being made.)

"I'm frustrated, too," admits Francis. "I'd like to have an agent—yesterday. But I'm sure if we grit our teeth and grind on we'll get something." Still, Francis acknowledges how uncertain the search for an unknown infective agent can be. "I have nightmares that the AIDS agent is something that we're missing. I worry that the electron microscopist is passing over those big spots on the slide, looking for tiny viruses. Are those spots the bacteria that cause AIDS?" (Researchers searched for seven years for the cause of Lyme arthritis, which turned out to be a spirochete, a large spiral bacterium carried by wood ticks.)

Others share the nightmare. Says Harold Jaffe: "It's possible that the agent could be sitting right here under our noses and we don't have the technology to find it." Marc Conant agrees that this is a possibility: "I think we're dealing with a new agent—sui generis—in the human population. If that is the case, isolation could be difficult."

And Other Possibilities

It is possible that none of the viral agents discussed at the NIH meeting will turn out to be the actual culprit. A whole succession of agents may have to be investigated along the road to discovery, and many physicians feel that a treatment may be found before the causative pathogen is identified. Also to be remembered is the proposition that viruses that kill people are maladjusted and that killing the host is, if nothing else, poor policy. Many viral illnesses sweep through susceptible populations, adapt, and disappear.

But others do not pass so easily, and by midsummer 1983 there seemed no reason to think AIDS would be so accommodating. So what are the possibilities of an epidemic? Based on experience with other epidemics, there are several.

Marcus Conant recalls a childhood in the South filled with the summer threat of polio. "At the beginning of the summer none of the kids had antibodies to polio. Then almost everyone was infected with the virus, and a few went on to get sick. The rest of us developed resistance. By the end of the summer most of the children would have antibodies."

An alternate scenario is suggested by Jon Gold. "Legionnaire's was a big mystery when it was first starting. People had wild ideas about what it could be. Was it a toxin, or a heavy-metal poison such as nickel? There were many speculations and all were valid because no one knew what it might be. Then a cause was found, and now we all understand it. Many unexplained epidemics turn out the same way; it's just that all the pieces finally fit together. AIDS may take the same course—or it may not.

"In the future, an apparently unrelated disease or some unrelated finding may give us the clue that will pull it all together, and against that day [Dr. Donald] Armstrong and I store as many specimens as possible. We can't yet find a virus. Maybe in twenty years someone will—in Australia or in gold miners in South Africa, and people will go back and test that serum against our samples and say, 'My God! This is AIDS!' "

The finding of the clusters of men with AIDS in 1981 pointed to an agent that was sexually transmitted. This finding initially seemed to clarify the confusing epidemiology of the new disease. "The most obvious thing would be that if it is sexually transmitted, here are examples of people who have given it to each other," says Harold Jaffe. "The alternative hypothesis, though, is a more complex one which makes you more cautious. It is that people who have sex with each other presumably have other things in common; they probably lead similar lives. It is possible that what we were seeing was simply a very small subgroup of homosexual men who did have sex with each other but that was not their true risk factor, that the true risk factor was drugs or something else that they also shared because their lives were very similar." But most researchers felt confident that AIDS was being transmitted by homosexual practices; the feeling gave them a marginal sense of forward progress. This was transitory. A new population was to enter the saga of AIDS, one that raised new issues and threw what had seemed to be solid leads back into question.

6

New Horizons

Misfortune
Wandering the same track
Lights now upon one and
Now upon another.
    —Aeschylus, *Prometheus Bound*

There were more than 36 million hospital admissions in the United States in 1981. Many were for routine surgery, many for chronic conditions. Babies were born, old people died, and millions of accidents and episodes of acute illness filled emergency rooms.

Against this noisy background it should be no surprise that the first cases of what might have been AIDS in Haitians went unnoticed in hospitals scattered across the country. In Jackson Memorial Hospital in Miami, the procession of critically ill Haitians at first attracted little attention.

"We were in the middle of the 'boat people,' " recalls young Dr. Margaret Fischl, "and I had just been appointed Associate Director of Medicine." Then came AIDS, and Fischl was introduced to a whole new phase of medicine, "where people flock to you and look up to you. I have difficulty dealing with my inability to help them.

"It's exciting to watch a whole new disease unfold," says the scientist in Fischl. But there is a price: "It's so time consuming. The patients never seem to stop coming in and some of them are so incredibly ill. You work around the clock, some get better and are discharged, and then they come back with another infection. It's so frustrating," she sighs.

But frustration and hard work alone would not take such a toll. Looking like an outlander among Miami's perpetually tanned residents, Fischl is white-skinned, her eyes ringed black by exhaustion. The price she is paying is also personal. Her attachment to the Haitian patients is evident and is reciprocated by their concern for her.

One of her first patients, a twenty-six-year-old divinity student, Destiné, first came in with toxoplasmosis; then he went on to contract a series of infections over the following months—PCP, candidiasis, cryptococcal meningitis, systemic CMV. With each new "symptom" of AIDS his ability to withstand illness diminished, and finally failed. In July 1983 Destiné died of overwhelming infection.

"He never once complained, but he was so disappointed every time he seemed to begin to recover—and then fell sick again. The few times he expressed his feelings about AIDS, he said it must be the will of God. He wasn't angry; he just asked me to help him get well and, if that wasn't possible, he'd accept that, too. He was always afraid I was going to get sick. He had a minister come in to baptize me so I'd stay well—physically and spiritually."

The Boat People

When the first Haitian AIDS patients began appearing at Jackson Memorial in May 1981, before the existence of the new immune-deficiency disease was common knowledge, none of the physicians could understand what might be wrong. "We really didn't know what to make of it," Fischl explains. "We couldn't put it together." Many of the Haitians were mal-nourished; most had had recent bouts of TB; almost all were young and recent immigrants—legal and illegal.

Even if the Miami physicians had known about the PCP in Los Angeles and the KS in New York, they would not have been likely to connect those outbreaks with what they were seeing. The Haitians were developing peculiar infections of the brain. Looking through his microscope at a snippet of brain tissue from one of the patients, Dr. George Hensley called on all he had learned in his twenty-two years as a pathologist. But there was no sense in what he was seeing. Although the young Haitian had been diagnosed as having TB of a particularly vicious nature, Hensley was far from satisfied that what he had under the microscope fit the disease. Perhaps it was an unusual form of TB; Hensley couldn't be sure. None of his colleagues could help, either. "It just didn't look right," he says.

Over the next few months, tissues from three more post-mortem cases that resembled the first one were accumulated in the laboratory freezer. All were from recently immigrated Haitians. Examining the last one, everything came clear: Hensley recognized the dark purple-stained beads of toxo-plasma gondii, a rarely found organism harbored by cats that occasionally causes death in premature infants.

"Toxoplasma has many forms in its life cycle. Most often in infected humans all you find is a tiny form that's very hard to see unless you're looking for it, which we weren't. But in that one case the organism was also present in a large, easily visualized form," Hensley explains.

"Once you know you're looking for toxo, it's very, very

easy to see, so we went into our 'files' and looked at the tissues from the first three cases—and sure enough, there were millions of toxoplasma gondii. Bang! We had an epidemic."

The appearance of AIDS in this unusual form emphasized the special aspect of the disease that made it extremely difficult to diagnose or identify during the first years of the disease. The compromised immune system allows a wide spectrum of organisms carried by the infected person to be turned loose to cause disease and death. In the newly immigrated Haitians, the public health conditions in their poor country have caused most of the population to carry infective organisms that have not been encountered by citizens of the industrialized countries in generations. Tuberculosis, for instance, which is seldom fatal in America anymore, is a leading cause of death in Haiti.

When the impoverished immigrants began appearing in the Miami hospital in 1979 with various complications of TB, doctors thought that the neurologic symptoms from which they suffered—confusion, seizures, disorientation—meant that the TB organism had reached the brain and was causing encephalitis. There seemed to be little reason to look beyond that until Hensley finally satisfied his gut feeling that "disseminated tuberculosis of the brain" was not an adequate diagnosis.

"The first patient whom we diagnosed correctly was in deep coma, but once we knew he was infected with toxo, we treated him properly, and he finally walked out of the hospital. To us it was a miracle," Hensley recalls. Most of the previous patients, undiagnosed, had died within fifteen days of admission to the hospital. Unfortunately, even the identification of toxoplasma as one of the infections did not mean that patients would recover. Like Destiné, they were rescued from one infection, only to succumb to another.

"Just after we diagnosed that first case of toxo a Public Health person called to inquire if we had seen any gay men with an immunosuppressive syndrome who were highly infected with CMV. 'Well,' I said, 'we don't have anything like that but we do have several Haitians who've died with toxo and CMV in their brains.' "

But gay men began to come in as well, and between the end of 1979 and the summer of 1982, there were twenty cases of AIDS in Miami. Nine men and one woman had died. The cost of caring for them at Jackson Memorial rose to $1.2 million.

Why Haitians?

By mid-1982 the epidemic of AIDS among Haitians was well established. Haitians were sickening and dying from the disease in New York, New Jersey, and Montreal. Some of these people were long-term U.S. residents; most were recent arrivals. Their possible risk factor was a complete mystery. All but one denied absolutely having had homosexual encounters or using IV drugs. "It was quite strange to us," says Dr. Hensley, "that this group of people did not share the risk factors." Even in early 1983, Margaret Fischl, shaking her head emphatically in the negative, said, "I can categorically state that the patients we have seen so far are heterosexual. Only one Haitian patient here has been homosexual."

If they weren't gay what was causing them to contract an illness virtually identical to the others with AIDS? Rumors of voodoo practices, of ritual scarring, of AIDS having been hidden away in the poverty-stricken island, circulated wildly. Seeking a new life in the United States, the Haitians were stigmatized by the past they were trying to escape.

In late 1982 a report of twelve cases of Kaposi's in Haiti had filtered out to the United States. Dr. Arthur Levine expressed the confusion of researchers when he said, "The fact that AIDS has only recently been diagnosed in Haiti doesn't mean it's something new on the island. It may be because there is now a dermatologist there who came from Africa a year ago where he'd seen Kaposi's sarcoma, so that when he got to Haiti, he knew what he was seeing. There might have been twelve cases a year for the last four hundred years in Haiti and no one would have known what it was.

"My intuition is that AIDS has long been endemic in Haiti," speculated Levine. "We would have no way of knowing about it because there is so much chronic illness, malnutrition, pneumonia, and early death there. And no oncologist would have recognized KS amid this background of illness. When the homosexuals started going there for vacations, interacting with the Haitians, it could have entered the homosexual bloodstream, as it were. But the obverse is also possible: the gays could have gone down there carrying the disease and introduced it into the Haitian population."

Amid the confusion, Hensley and his chief resident, Lee Moskowitz, flew to Haiti to attempt to gather some facts. "When you are faced with an insoluble problem," Hensley says, "you always fall back on a historical perspective. It was possible that the disease was being caused by a virus that was not new, that AIDS was endemic somewhere in the world and had recently entered a new population. We surmised it might be endemic on the island. That was a familiar hypothesis and that makes you more comfortable—it explains what you don't know."

But Hensley's hope was short-lived. In Port-au-Prince, the capital city, the doctors were allowed to look through pathology archives of the past several years at three hospitals that represented a cross section of the socioeconomic strata of the country. Of the first trip, in June 1982, Moskowitz says,

"We found that there were diseases like AIDS. I found a case of KS. And there were unexplained deaths from things like candida, PCP, CMV."

A month later the pathologists returned to Haiti for a more thorough search. They used the diagnosis of TB of the brain as their clue to possible AIDS. "We had seen confusion between TB encephalitis and CNS toxo at Jackson Memorial," reasoned Hensley, "so we looked at cases of TB in Haiti to try to find toxo, which could have been a marker disease for AIDS. And we looked for other diseases—leukemia, lymphoma.

"We found a number of AIDS-like cases, but as we traced back in time they became fewer. Our oldest documented case was in October 1978. Previous to that there were only a few suspicious histories and no cases that we could call AIDS.

"The upshot of the whole thing is that we found that AIDS had started at about the same time in Haiti as it did in the U.S. So it is no more likely that the disease was imported into this country from Haiti than vice versa."

"There's nothing that tells us that the Haitians are the cause of the disease," adds Dr. Moskowitz. "Or that American gays are the cause of the disease in Haiti. It probably started somewhere else and arrived in the U.S. and Haiti simultaneously."

The Island in the Sun

The telephone call that had alerted Jackson Memorial doctors to the developing AIDS epidemic—into which their Haitian patients would soon be reluctantly added—also alerted the CDC to the existence of a potential new risk group. Their first "quick and dirty" nine-city phone survey had turned up something in the Haitian cases that no one could have predicted.

Dr. Harry Haverkos, CDC epidemiologist, was in it from the beginning. He found both "serendipitous" good fortune and almost insurmountable stumbling blocks to the inclusion of the Haitians in the epidemic. Taking a week off from the second case-control study of AIDS patients, Haverkos went to Miami. Examining the autopsy records at Jackson Memorial, he says, "I saw the unusual toxoplasma infections, some PCP, and that their immune systems were even more depressed than those of the gay men. But I wasn't sure it was the same disease. There was a lot of TB and many of the patients were cachectic [malnourished and wasted].

"I talked to an anthropologist who had worked with Haitians, to some Haitian social workers, and attempted to talk to family members of those who had died. Basically, I found out nothing. I wasn't convinced that we were asking the right questions or that what we were asking was in the proper cultural context."

The good fortune was a vacation trip to Haiti made by EIS officer, Dr. Alain Rosin, who had worked on the island with the World Health Organization before joining CDC. While in Haiti, Rosin met a Dr. Liataud, the dermatologist from Africa to whom Dr. Levine had referred. At that time, Liataud had diagnosed nine cases of KS in Haiti. Says Dr. Haverkos: "So we found out firsthand that there was something going on in Haiti that met the CDC case definition of AIDS."

Something certainly was. To George Hensley it smacked of a public health problem: "I personally believe that in Haiti it's a water-borne disease. Believe me," says Hensley, "the water supply of Haiti is badly contaminated."

Hensley's conjecture is entirely his own, but all manner

of epidemiological straws were being grasped. As late as mid-1983, Jon Gold of Sloan-Kettering said, "This is wild speculation, but . . . I'm very interested in exotic viruses and one we haven't looked at is the one that causes hemorrhagic swine fever. This virus is endemic in Haiti. It causes immuno-suppression in swine and low white-blood-cell counts, and has a very high mortality rate. In fact, they're killing all the pigs in Haiti to get rid of the epizootic."

There were more exotic notions. Death from contaminated instruments used in voodoo rites or decorative scarring, "drinking" blood, evil spirits, and witch doctors were all put forth as possible explanations of the etiology of AIDS. But those speculations underlined the fact that Americans are basically uninformed about the realities of life in this island republic.

Haiti is a country of roughly 5.5 million people with an average yearly income of less than $100 per capita. What wealth there is is in the hands of the small, educated elite. Of the citizens of Haiti, 90 percent are illiterate; of Haiti's $1.2 billion gross national product, $80 million comes in through the tourist trade. Amnesty International has called the Haitian government "the most repressive in the western hemisphere," and this apparently was exacerbated when Jean-Claude (Bébé Doc) Duvalier succeeded his father to the Presidency-for-Life. At that time, the mid-1970s, the Haitian exodus speeded up; presently, about 6 percent of all Haitians are expatriated. Those who were illegal immigrants were already in an unenviable situation. AIDS has created sheer panic.

The health of the Haitian population still on the island is "severely compromised by infections and inadequate nutrition," according to Dr. Jean-Claude Compas, of the Haitian Medical Association Abroad in New York. No one knows—

and many say no one cares—precisely what are the infections that kill so many Haitians.

Compounding a Problem

As gay men feel they are being "blamed" for AIDS, Haitians also feel persecuted; they feel they are falsely labeled as a disease-carrying national group. Their early reluctance to answer questions, according to Dr. Fischl, was "due to the fact that everything they said was met with skepticism. To immediately say they're not telling the truth is irresponsible, biased. It was very demeaning to the Haitians and they were insulted by that. It made them leery of cooperating."

For many Haitians—having left a country in which they were afraid to say what they thought, and having become ill with a deadly disease—being questioned in a foreign tongue, often by medical officials of the government that could ship them back to Haiti, was a terrifying experience. Moreover, the acts about which they were being questioned are taboo in their own country. The Reverend Jean Juste, a spokesman for the Miami Haitian community, has accused the Reagan administration of "playing a political game through AIDS toward Haitians," presumably to stop them from remaining in America.

Certainly, since AIDS was found among them, the Haitian lot in the United States has been a poor one. As a "risk group," all Haitians are perceived as being carriers of the disease. They have lost jobs and housing, and their children have been ostracized.

"Who knows if a man is homosexual?" asks a Haitian cab driver in New York. "I am black and speak with a French accent. For that, my children are not allowed to play with children in school. Now I say I am from Martinique," the man ended bitterly.

"Identifying them as a group has caused Haitians considerable hardship," Dr. Haverkos admits. "We and the people in the New York City Health Department have gotten numerous questions about whether it's safe to have Haitians working in hotels and restaurants." (Their answer: Yes.)

The Haitian response to being classified as a group at risk has swung from an initial denial of there being any AIDS in Haiti to denial that being Haitian constitutes a risk per se. Haitians living in this country have attacked the CDC for naming the entire national group and have claimed that the epidemiology to back that claim is faulty and insubstantial.

This has angered many at CDC. "It's really insulting for people to say that we're making mistakes because we don't know how to do epidemiology," Harold Jaffe bristles. "I wouldn't go into an operating room and tell someone how much anesthesia to use, and I don't see where they get the idea that it's any different in my discipline."

As director of the CDC during the first two years of the AIDS investigation, Dr. William Foege says, "I've thought about this, about what we could have done differently. It's an overriding belief of mine that when you tangle with culture, culture wins. But, having said that, I also believe you don't dilute or distort your science, even if it causes problems. So when we found certain groups at risk, we had to make it known. It would have been indefensible to cloud that over.

"The problem is that there has been too much confusion over what 'high risk' means. It means they are at risk of getting the disease. Gays and Haitians are *not* a risk to you and me. Perhaps we should have done something to make sure that no one discriminated against gays or Haitians. I wish I knew how to really solve that problem." The touchiness of the CDC over the Haitian dilemma caused the usually composed Jim

Curran to mishear and angrily reply to a writer's question during a New York AIDS Conference in November 1983. Asked what plans were being made to avoid the problems that have been encountered in questioning Haitians once the CDC participates in epidemiology in Africa, Curran snapped, "You members of the press are responsible for the discrimination against the Haitians!" The question that was asked was repeated; no answer was forthcoming.

Foege thinks that not all Haitians are equally at risk. "We know the risk is real in Haitians, and we think it may be much higher in those who have come to the U.S. in the past five years. But we don't yet know the demographics." In Miami, the incidence of AIDS is greater than one per thousand Haitians—almost as great as among gays in New York.

The Massisi

Finally, in spring 1983, the Haitian government and the Haitian Medical Society assigned a risk factor to Haitians with AIDS: they were men who had engaged in male prostitution. At a May meeting in Haiti, data was presented from three studies that claimed to show that various percentages of male AIDS patients in the country admitted to homosexual contact. Why had not the CDC picked up on this? Because, asserted Reverend Juste and other Haitian leaders, they lacked the expertise to conduct epidemiological surveys in another language and among people from another culture.

Dr. Compas, who also heads the Haitian Coalition on AIDS, was infuriated that an entire national group had been singled out. "For Haitians, being named a 'risk group' seems like a politically motivated slur. Haitians with AIDS have the identical risk factors as any of those at risk. Because of the poverty in Haiti, young men prostitute themselves for money. This is very common, but they would never call themselves homosexuals. And they would be insulted if you called them that.

"What is different is that these *massisi* [the Haitian word for male homosexual] are also married and infect their wives or girlfriends." On a recent trip to Haiti, Compas spoke to the women who had contracted AIDS. "All of them had husbands or boyfriends who had been very sick or had died during the past six months," he said.

Dr. Ary Bordes, Haitian Minister of Health, is of the opinion that AIDS has been introduced into Haiti by American gays. He expressed the Haitian government's official position by stating that "most AIDS in Haiti is in places where the tourists come." Dr. Bordes also suggested that paramedical people "set themselves up as doctors and give shots with dirty needles." Asked about the large number of Haitian women with AIDS—one-third of cases on the island—Bordes said it was "because of sodomy." (Anal intercourse is common in countries where either the money to purchase prophylactic devices or the knowledge of other birth-control measures is lacking.)

The Haitian Ministry has undertaken their own epidemiological study from which they expect "to get the truth and firmly assign AIDS risk to promiscuous gays," according to Bordes.

This "finding" was widely proclaimed as a solution to the Haitian AIDS mystery by the American press. Newly arrived from a visit to Port-au-Prince, TV science correspondent Bob Bazell stated in an article in the August 1, 1983, *New Republic*:

> There is simply no evidence to support the so-called "Haitian connection." When Haitian doctors interviewed the victims, they learned that at least one-quarter had worked as male prostitutes meeting foreign gay men, mostly

Americans, in bars in Port-au-Prince and in the resort areas of Cap Haitien. These Haitian men did not consider themselves homosexual. In fact, there is a strong cultural taboo against homosexuality in Haiti. Many of these men were married with families. They had sold themselves in order to survive.

Dr. Joyce Johnson, a CDC task force member, attended the meeting in Haiti where the three studies were presented, and her impression was that "it was not clear, because of the various survey methods used, exactly how many of the Haitian AIDS cases are homosexual or bisexual. I'd guess at most 10 percent of their AIDS cases were explained by homosexual contact."

But the data fit with the Haitian government's policies. A few months after the sexual preferences of AIDS patients in Haiti were widely proclaimed in the press, authorities in Port-au-Prince, in what many called a "cosmetic gesture," raided a gay hotel and bar. The government then announced that all homosexual men would be jailed for six months, and spend six more months in "rehabilitation." Evidently, a number of prominent gays who were scooped up in the raid threatened to "name names," and all were quickly released.

Dr. Bordes said that foreigners who owned gay establishments were asked to leave the country at once.

Trying for the Truth
In August 1983, a meeting with Haitian leaders was held in Atlanta with CDC personnel and two of the physicians who have seen the most cases among Haitians, Drs. Fischl of Miami and Sheldon Landesman of Brooklyn. The task was to enlist the aid of the Haitian professionals in drawing up a questionnaire that would have more success potential in defining which Haitian nationals were or were not at risk for AIDS.

(At this meeting more than 150 cases were estimated on the island, and, according to Dr. Adrian Marcel, a Haitian doctor now working in New York, "the hospitals are loaded with those dying from diarrhea," a frequent symptom of AIDS. A more realistic estimate may be in excess of 300 cases [as reported six months later by Haitian doctors]. Although it's difficult to enumerate accurately, since reporting protocols have changed, Haitian nationals represent about 5.5 percent of U.S. AIDS cases.)

In a small, windowless room, for the better part of a day, Drs. Jaffe and Johnson went question by question through the twenty-page document that Johnson had devised as a starting point. During this procedure a profile of Haiti's sexual mores was gradually elicited.

"If you're white, you can't step outside your Holiday Inn in Port-au-Prince and not be swarmed over by ten boys between the ages of ten and sixteen years," said Haitian businessman Yves Savain, and former head of the Miami Haitian Task Force. "They will start by offering you a woman, then drugs, then anything else you might want—including themselves. Gay bars are very recent; that's a phenomenon that has only existed for the past five years or so."

Dr. Fischl, who had earlier been convinced that her Haitian patients had not participated in gay sex, spoke of the problems she had encountered in obtaining detailed information: "I ask if they have had oral or rectal sex—and the answer is yes or no. But when I've asked, 'Have you ever inserted your penis in another person's mouth?' they've either been horrified—or laughed."

Fischl also related the history of one of her patients who had four children, all under five years old, "by different wives, none of whom he lived with." Savain replied that it was not unusual in Miami, as "having a child is the way the mother can be assured of not being kicked out of the United States. So a man who gets a reputation for fathering children may be much sought after."

Questions regarding the status of nutrition and sanitation in Haiti were included in the questionnaire, as well as queries about the movements of Haitians since their arrival in this country. "That's very important," Fischl reminded the group. "You need to know whether they've been back, or had visitors from Haiti, when they came, etcetera."

Landesman brought up several concerns about the general health condition of the Haitian population. The incidence of both malaria and malnutrition on the island have given rise to questions pertaining to the immune depression caused by these conditions. But half of the world's population suffers from the effects of hunger; and probably 200,000 new cases of malaria are reported each year. These are permanent, chronic problems in all underdeveloped countries. The likelihood that they impact on AIDS is remote.

Harold Jaffe wanted to know if the kind of prostitution practiced in Haiti was also found in the United States, and Savain replied: "Most likely. To keep a job in Miami, the employee is sometimes expected to have sex with the owner."

The conclusion of the long overdue consultation was that there are many questions necessary to obtain valid answers from Haitians surveyed. (Is sex for pleasure? for money? etc.) Dr. Marcel, who volunteers in several New York area clinics that treat his countrymen, suggested that Haitian doctors might not be able to ascertain honest information. "One of our patients in New Jersey, who had been in this country for ten months, had severe diarrhea, lymphadenopathy, and a 'wart' on his penis on which they were going to operate," Marcel recounted. "We suspected AIDS and sent him to Dr. Friedman-Kien. The 'wart' was Kaposi's. The man was married, with two children, and denied ever having sex with a man. It took five months for him to admit that he had—in Haiti— just to make some money.

"But that's what you'd expect. To be homosexual in Haiti is very taboo. It really is not safe. There is no justice in Haiti, no law, nothing absolute. It is a dictatorship with a head who is as smart as my left foot and who is and always has been rumored to himself be gay." (Duvalier is also said to be suffering from lupus, an autoimmune disease unusual in men and said by Arthur Levine to be a possible manifestation of AIDS.)

Given all the complexities, it has been impossible to get a clear fix on the magnitude of AIDS in Haiti. And from at least a semblance of cooperation with American investigators, the official climate has changed. Hensley says, "Since we went to Haiti, apparently cooperation has decreased. They say the identification of Haitians as a risk group for AIDS has had an effect on tourism."

Unfortunately, the validity of AIDS data coming from Haiti has to be questioned. The consequences of a large number of cases of AIDS, most of which cannot be assigned to homosexual activity, easily could mean the death of the tourist business on which the country's marginal finances depend. Dr. Bordes further threw into doubt the official reporting practice of his Ministry of Health. Responding to a question asked by *The New York Times* in an interview on August 16, 1983, Bordes said, "Scientifically I have no reluctance to provide the information [to the CDC]. But if those data will destroy my country, I will not do it because my main duty is to my country."

Even as the initial steps in the joint study were being taken, evidence appeared indicating that AIDS in Haitians could not be satisfactorily explained by homosexuality. In the *New England Journal of Medicine* of October 20, 1983, an article was published entitled "Characteristics of the Acquired Immunodeficiency Syndrome (AIDS) in Haiti." It contained data from a cooperative study conducted by Dr. Warren D. Johnson, Jr., of Cornell University Medical College and the Haitian Study Group on Kaposi's sarcoma and opportunistic infection in Haiti. The Haitian doctors included Dr. Bernard Liataud, the physician who had identified the first cases of Kaposi's sarcoma among Haitians in Haiti. In this study, conducted by Haitian physicians speaking to patients in their native language and cognizant of the local customs, only 15 percent of the male AIDS patients admitted to having "sexual activity with both men and women." Even among patients pointedly questioned about sexual practices by a member of the Haitian AIDS Study Group only 24 percent admitted to bisexuality. Thus, 75 percent or more of the cases of AIDS among male Haitians remained unexplained.

African Genesis?

While Haitians were joining the ranks of AIDS victims in Miami, New York, New Jersey, and Montreal, doctors at a hospital in Saint Antoine, France, were attempting to treat a young African woman, the wife of a diplomat recently arrived from Zaire. Twenty-three years old and previously healthy, between June 1981 and her death in March 1982 she suffered from a succession of infectious illnesses that included PCP, mycobacterium, and salmonella. Her abnormal T-cell ratio, the absence of lymphocytes, and anergy to skin tests marked her as a classic case of AIDS.

Speculation on an African linkage for AIDS has circulated from the early days of the illness. Kaposi's sarcoma is an important and deadly disease on that continent; Burkitt's lymphoma, thought to be caused in part by the EBV so common in gay men, was identified in East Africa; many of the diarrheas and infections of AIDS seem remarkably analogous to African disorders.

But by what route, through what connection, could a pathogen have been transferred from Africa to North America? One theory was put forward by Dr. Caroline MacLeod, director of the University of Miami's Tropical Diseases laboratory. MacLeod speculated that Cuban soldiers returning from Angola brought the virus that subsequently spread through contact with Haitians. (Other researchers discounted this idea, citing the fact that there was no evidence of AIDS in Cuba.)

A more direct and plausible route may be the close connection between the French-speaking countries of Haiti and what once was the Belgian Congo—now Zaire. When Zaire became independent from its colonial overseer, Belgium, and began setting up its own infrastructure, Haitian nationals were contracted to fill many positions as teachers, managers, bureaucrats.

This was in the early 1960s, and over the years, Haitians traveled back and forth between the two countries on home leaves and vacations. Dr. Compas says that many Haitians are still in Zaire and that many who completed their contracts returned to the United States—not Haiti.

Dan William says this is his "pet theory"; and the sequence of events would appear to substantiate such a connection. This theory suggests the possibility of an infectious agent carried by a near-identical genetic pool without a need to transform itself into a more lethal pathogen.

When the longtime dictator of Haiti, Papa Doc Duvalier, died in the early 1970s, tourism from the States began in earnest, and gay men, particularly New Yorkers, made it their "place in the sun," according to Dr. Larry Puchall of Washington, D.C. If the time sequence is correct—and given a suspected incubation period of up to three years—a different, white genetic group was brought into contact with the infective agent.

"It was an easy step from Haiti to the gay community in the United States by virtue of gay men on vacation," William says. But as neatly as this theory fits Africa–Haiti–New York into an answer to the question of where the agent came from, there are still loose ends. For example: has an AIDS-like disease been seen in equatorial Africa before? Dr. Charles Olweny of Uganda, who for many years was associated with the then-prestigious Makerere University Medical School and hospital in Kampala, states unequivocally that he never saw illnesses in Africans that fulfilled the CDC criteria for AIDS. And other physicians with African experience agree.

Furthermore, such a theory does little to explain the sudden rash of cases among Zairian and Chad nationals in Belgium and France, none of which have interacted with Americans or Haitians of any sexual inclinations. In France, nine AIDS cases were diagnosed prior to summer 1981, and several of these were in white Frenchmen who had lived or traveled extensively in central Africa and had no contact with the United States or Haiti.

In November 1983, the World Health Organization issued a report on the international incidence of AIDS indicating that the disease is indeed a worldwide problem, with cases in thirty-three countries and all inhabited continents. Lawrence Altman, reporting on the WHO conference in Geneva where the findings were announced, wrote in *The New York Times*: "Of particular concern is a spurt in cases diagnosed in Europe, where the number has doubled in the last year. . . . And there are indications that in Africa the disease may be striking heterosexual men and women in equal numbers. . . . Despite the small number of cases reported in some countries, many participants said they suspected the true incidence of AIDS was more widespread than believed. They said the incidence of AIDS might be many times greater than the official worldwide total. . . ."

Belgium reports forty cases (of which 40 percent are women), all related in some way to central Africa, according to Dr. Jan Desmyter of the Riga Institute in Louvain. Desmyter also suggested that there may have been AIDS in Zaire "ten or twenty years ago." In Kinshasa, Zaire, more than one thousand cases have been seen.

In the large African population of Paris, twenty people have contracted the disease. France has more than one hundred cases overall, with the number doubling every six months, according to Dr. J. B. Brunet of the Ministry of Health.

Natives of the African countries of Gabon, Mali, Rwanda, Cameroon, and Burundi have also been diagnosed with AIDS in Europe.

If epidemiologists have a difficult time accumulating accurate information from Haiti and Europe, the prodigious task of going into Africa's vast, largely isolated, and illiterate population would appear near impossible. We may never know where AIDS had its genesis.

Dr. Fischl is not optimistic about AIDS remaining confined to any present risk group. "If AIDS is a sexually transmitted disease, as all evidence indicates, then it will spread to the general population—although homosexuals will remain at higher risk for contracting it," Fischl states. "We will see it spread through the heterosexual community, and ten years from now it will be just like hepatitis B—anyone will be able to get it, few will."

7

Blood and Needles

Present fears
are less than horrible imaginings.
—Shakespeare,
Macbeth

For a recreational shooter in the Bronx, it is safest to do drugs in a "shooting gallery": a hole-in-the-wall apartment or the still-intact portion of an abandoned building. In that way, if stopped by the police on the street, they aren't holding drugs or the paraphernalia used to inject them. Hardcore junkies occasionally use the galleries, but it is primarily weekend users who congregate there.

"These aren't 'wild-eyed drug fiends,' " says Dr. Gerald Friedland, Associate Professor of Medicine at Albert Einstein Medical Center in the Bronx. "They use drugs the same way our culture uses alcohol; it's a social event, a get-together. Many of my patients have marginal jobs and live in crowded apartments with several generations together in a few rooms."

But the social habit of injecting drugs into their bloodstreams has introduced another element into often already desperate lives. It has brought AIDS. The effect of this, says Friedland, is "devastating."

The South Bronx is a poor, colorful world. Two-thirds of the New York borough's 1.5 million population is of Hispanic extraction, and of these, two-thirds are Puerto Rican. While this mixed culture is producing many successful citizens, there is still great poverty and social dislocation for those who live in the tenements of the Bronx.

Shooting galleries provide a kind of social environment, a clublike setting. There drugs are bought and needles and other equipment are rented to users who cook up heroin, draw it into a syringe, and inject it into a muscle or vein. The syringe—which costs about $2 to rent for each injection—is put down, to be reused by as many as forty to seventy others until the needle is too dull to penetrate skin. No thought is given to assuring that the needle, or the skin into which it will go, is clean. In this fashion, hepatitis has been spread through the drug-using population; it now appears that AIDS may be spreading by the same route.

The first cases of PCP in IV drug abusers were reported in December 1981, from New York City, along with several cases in male homosexuals. At that time the scope of the epidemic was not appreciated, nor did those doctors mention transmission by blood or needles. As Harold Jaffe says, "When we first got the reports on the IV drug users we didn't really know what to make of them. I think they were all dead at the time they were reported, and we thought, well, maybe there is a common drug usage between the homosexuals and IV drug users."

But as time went on and the number of AIDS patients who were not homosexuals but were IV drug abusers stabilized at 17 percent, spread of the illness via contaminated needles began to be considered more closely. "Ultimately we did twenty or thirty interviews with IV drug abusers who had AIDS," Jaffe recounts. "We learned that these people did not use nitrites much and they were not particularly sexually active. It probably was the thing that really got us thinking that if we are dealing with an infectious disease, then it was one for which hepatitis B was a model." (Hepatitis B is a viral illness spread primarily via blood.)

While AIDS was alarming New York and the West Coast cities of Los Angeles and San Francisco, in Miami a hemophiliac was dying of an opportunistic infection—finally diagnosed as AIDS. Between the hemophiliacs and intravenous drug users lay a common bond—needles and blood. And AIDS took on another dimension. "We learned about the first case of AIDS in a hemophiliac in January 1982," says Dr. Bruce Evatt of CDC. "He was a fifty-five-year-old man in Miami who came down with a pneumonia. The doctors diagnosed pneumocystis, which surprised them since they hadn't seen this organism in their hospital. They thought it was due to contamination of the man's Factor VIII."

By the time the CDC heard of this case, the man was dead. Two roadblocks stood in the way of a firm diagnosis of AIDS: no thorough studies of his immune system had been done, and the patient had been treated with steroids, which are themselves immunosuppressive. "We flagged the pentamidine file," Evatt recalls. "Dr. Foege said, 'If this is real there will be another case and another.' And in June and July we had our next two cases, one in Ohio and one in Colorado."

Up to this point sexual transmission between gay men had been identified as the only route by which AIDS traveled from person to person. The finding of the clusters had strengthened this theory. But blood had not been put completely aside: anal intercourse often is "a bloody business," as one researcher had remarked, and breaks in the fragile rectal mucosa were suspected to be entry points for an infective agent.

Many other factors had been ruled out or pushed to one side; poppers and pathogens in bathhouses were unlikely causes, particularly in view of the occurrences of AIDS in Haitians. The introduction of a new viral agent was attracting the most attention, though many still clung to the "overload" theory. A combination of the two—a new agent attacking people already carrying multiple infections—was also thought a possible scenario for AIDS susceptibility.

Finding drug abusers and hemophiliacs with AIDS did little to steer these possibilities in a single direction. Both groups were known to be exposed to a multitude of infectious organisms. Those who shoot illegal drugs are almost universally infected with hepatitis B, EBV, CMV, and other infections. Hemophiliacs also inject themselves, some as many as eight times a week, to prevent dangerous bleeding. Though hemophiliacs use sterile equipment and are careful to avoid infection, the material they require to remain healthy carries multiple unwanted substances.

Hemophilia

Out of every 100,000 people in the American population, two or three are hemophiliacs. This inherited blood-clotting disorder is passed in the female X chromosome by mothers to their male offspring. When hemophilia is carried in a family line, girl babies have a 50:50 chance of inheriting from their mothers a defective X chromosome. Since a female has two X chromosomes, however, one X will be healthy and prevent hemophilia. If a male infant—who has only one X—inherits the defective one from his mother, he is a hemophiliac. Hemophilia can be mild or severe depending on the degree of the lack of the clotting substance known as Factor VIII.

Hemophilia can cause death from bleeding from a cut; it also causes severe pain and joint damage because of small bleeders deep within the tissues. In past years most males with hemophilia died young and surgery was unthinkable. Effective treatment for this disease was first developed in the 1960s.

One product used in treating hemophilia, cryoprecipitate (cryo), is made from the blood serum of a single normal donor. This is frozen and injected as needed to prevent bleeding. Cryo must be administered by a physician. The other preventive, Factor VIII concentrate, is made from the pooled donations of as many as 2,500 to 5,000 donors, quick-dried, and kept by the hemophiliac, who adds liquid and injects himself when bleeding episodes occur.

Both of these products are treated with chemicals and other means to kill pathogens carried in donor blood. Still, not all organisms are destroyed, so there is a calculated risk in these lifesaving substances. Since some with hemophilia need as many as forty vials a year to control bleeding, those using convenient Factor VIII concentrate are exposed to the blood of as many as 200,000 different people annually.

Treatment with Factor VIII, for this reason, has long been worrisome to some physicians. Dr. Oscar Ratnoff of Case Western Reserve Medical School in Cleveland, has said, "You can't expect to go on exposing people to protein from tens of thousands of strange people and get away with it for too long." Ratnoff and Dr. Jay Menitove of the Council of Community Blood Centers had both found changes in the T-cell ratios of hemophiliacs using Factor VIII.

Their individual papers in a medical journal had reported

that more than half the healthy hemophiliacs tested had reversed T-cell ratios similar to, but less severe than, those gay men with AIDS. These ratio reversals were found primarily in patients treated with Factor VIII; cryo recipients largely had normal ratio results.

Why Factor VIII?

Given the risks that come with exposure to so many foreign bloods, why would doctors and patients feel Factor VIII concentrate is nevertheless so desirable? Dr. David Aronson, a blood expert at the FDA, says that Factor VIII "has permitted hemophiliacs to lead relatively normal lives. During the period from 1968—when Factor VIII was developed—to 1979, the life expectancy of hemophiliacs has risen dramatically, from thirty-five to fifty-five years. It also allows them to undergo surgery and has greatly improved the quality of their lives."

Alan Brownstein, executive director of the National Hemophilia Foundation, makes a strong case in economic terms: "With this treatment, hospital care is down by more than 80 percent; the average number of days per year in hospitals is down from 9.4 to 1.8; the percent of unemployment in adults is down from 36 percent to 12.8 percent; and there is a reduction of 62 percent in total health-care costs per patient."

But, as Brownstein added, "It is ironic that the very substance that has served to liberate hemophiliacs from the disabling effects of the disease is now highly suspect as the source of AIDS in them." Dr. Jane Desforges, in an editorial in the *New England Journal of Medicine*, wrote, "Preventing the complications of the present treatment [AIDS] may take precedence over preventing the complications of hemophilia itself." (Subsequently, a California blood product company was forced to recall 16 lots [64,000 doses] of Factor VIII because a man in Austin, Texas, who was a frequent "donor" had died of AIDS. He had given blood fifty times over the preceding eleven months and had failed to identify himself as belonging to a risk group.)

Hemophiliacs were left with little room to maneuver. Their choices—forgoing treatment and risking bleeding to death, returning to the costs and time required to use cryo (which is not presently in abundant supply), or contracting a deadly disease.

On December 10, 1982, *MMWR* reported five more cases of AIDS in hemophiliacs. That same issue of *MMWR* detailed a case of AIDS with even more frightening implications: an infant had apparently acquired AIDS through a blood transfusion.

The infant was cared for and diagnosed by Dr. Arthur Ammann, then a specialist in pediatric infectious diseases at the University of California, San Francisco, Medical Center and now with Genetech. "The baby was born prematurely," Dr. Ammann says. "And he had Rh complications and other problems of prematurity. He received six transfusions during the first four days of life, and a number of other infusions of blood, platelets, and red cells over the next two weeks. At seven months the infant's problems started showing up. He got severe otitis media. Then oral candidiasis. At nine months of age he stopped eating and showed signs of liver damage.

"Shortly after his first birthday we tested the baby's immune function. It was abnormal. Soon after he got an atypical mycobacterium infection.

"The blood donors were traced by Dr. Selma Dritz and Dr. Herbert Perkins," recounts Dr. Ammann. "One was found to be a homosexual man who developed AIDS about eight months after donating the blood that went to the infant. We think he was infectious at the time he donated and that his blood was the source of the baby's AIDS."

This was the background behind the convening of a CDC blood meeting in Atlanta in January 1983. The incidence of AIDS in hemophiliacs was the prime reason for the meeting being called, but a far broader question was at issue. There are about 15,000 severe hemophiliacs in the United States; but there are more than three million transfusions a year of blood and blood products. Did AIDS in hemophiliacs and drug abusers, and especially the death of the San Francisco infant, mean that the AIDS agent had also invaded the nation's general blood supply?

The Business of Blood

We generally tend to think of blood for transfusions being donated by civic-minded citizens and being collected by Red Cross personnel and volunteers. In truth, blood is a huge, profit-making business in America.

About half of the millions of collected blood units do come through voluntary, nonprofit agencies. This donated blood largely is in the form of whole blood and is transfused in that form. The other half, according to Dr. Bruce Voeller of the National Gay Task Force, "is commercially collected from people of suspect health who need quick cash." Eighty percent of the world supply of plasma—the liquid fraction from which red blood cells have been removed—is collected in the United States in this fashion. From plasma, Factor VIII and many other products are made.

The making of Factor VIII is conducted by for-profit "plasmapheresis" centers, which in 1982 did $182 million in business. In these centers, paid donors are hooked to a pheresis machine that separates and retains the plasma, and returns the red blood cells along with fluids. The collected plasma, rich in a variety of materials, is used to produce many needed blood-derived products, among them gamma globulin and clotting factors.

These commercial interests represented another factor concerned with the possibility of a contaminated blood supply.

The Gay Stake in the Blood Supply

The gay community was in the no-win situation of being the major victim of AIDS and the population most likely to be carrying the unknown agent, and at the same time being stigmatized as having "bad blood."

From the most primitive to the most sophisticated mind, blood is perceived as far more than a vehicle by which oxygen and other essential elements are transported. Blood is life: it symbolizes magic powers, health, courage, lineage. From the Blood of the Lamb, which caused the Angel of Death to bypass the firstborn of the Jews, to the Communion wine representing the Blood of Christ, to pacts sealed in blood; from "good," "bad," and "blue," to hot and cold—blood expresses the human condition.

For gays, struggling for social acceptance and civil rights, the issue of blood—*their* blood—was multifaceted. Leaders agreed that blood donations should be avoided by any person at risk for AIDS. What was not agreed, however, was the method by which this could be effected. "If you adopt the policy of exclusion of all gays, you'll stigmatize at the time of a major civil-rights movement a group of whom only a tiny fraction qualify as the problem we are here to address," Voeller told the assembled meeting in Atlanta. Once again, the medical and social issues of AIDS were inextricably linked.

The "Horrible" Meeting at CDC

In the tangle of opinions and interests represented at the CDC that January, several items on the agenda had to be clarified:

• *Were hemophiliacs contracting AIDS through their clotting-factor medications? And, if so, through both cryo and Factor VIII?* Those representing hemophiliacs and the plasma industry wanted to make sure that an uninterrupted supply was available and uncontaminated.

• *Was there a possibility that the entire national blood pool might be in danger of carrying the AIDS agent?* Nonprofit whole-blood collection interests demurred on that point; sufficient evidence of such, they insisted, simply was not in. CDC task force members disagreed. Though slight, the possibility of such contamination needed to be acted on at once, in their opinions.

• *If exclusion of those at risk for AIDS were to be set in motion, how would such a policy be implemented?* Gay concerns were that there be no labeling of the homosexuals of the country per se.

The first question was posed by Dr. Bruce Evatt of the CDC task force: Could the meeting reach a consensus about how AIDS was affecting hemophiliacs? "Despite the fact that most hemophiliac deaths during the past five years were caused by bleeding disorders (42 percent), all [hemophiliac] deaths from AIDS have occurred in this past year," Evatt reported.

Jim Curran added to this information by stating that "about 74 hemophiliacs die each year. In 1982 there were 10 cases of AIDS in this group—and a 10 percent increase in fatal illness."

(By the time congressional hearings were held in August 1983, Brownstein would report that "one of every 300 severe hemophiliacs has contracted AIDS to this date.")

Suggestions from many quarters were made for further

studies before any action was taken, but the CDC pressed for a decision at once. "To bury our heads in the sand and say, 'Let's wait for more cases' is not an adequate public health measure," insisted Dr. Jeffrey Koplan. And Don Francis added, "The same process of doubt arose when AIDS was first suspected in other groups. The disease has a long latent period. We can't constantly react and be constantly behind the eight ball! How many cases of AIDS in hemophiliacs is enough before we recognize a problem and take some action?" (A new nonblood product to treat those with moderate hemophilia is being developed and clinically tested. The drug, DDAVP, developed as an antidiuretic for diabetes, is cheaper and carries no risk of carrying the "trash" that Factor VIII does.)

But the CDC's demand for action by no means suited most participants at the meeting. Reports of a few possible deaths due to transfusions of whole blood were not convincing arguments to Dr. Joseph Bove of Yale University, representing the American Association of Blood Banks. "We want to take all these sweeping measures just because one baby got AIDS after transfusion from a person who later came down with AIDS—and there *may* be a *few* other cases!" Bove exclaimed in disbelief.

And representatives of hemophiliacs had their own worries. "There is great concern about any action that would remove commercial concentrates from availability," explained Charles Carmen, chairman of the Hemophilia Foundation.

"Action" also carried unacceptable implications to immunologist Roger Enlow, representing the American Association of Physicians for Human Rights. "This problem is indelibly etched on the consciousness of the homosexual community. So any kind of communication for voluntary cooperation will be heeded. But to continue to enjoy our goodwill and cooperation you really could not start a labeling process.

We are against any screening method that requires people to identify themselves on the basis of sexual preference," Enlow stated firmly.

This was, indeed, the social issue that had to be addressed. Like questions put to Haitians, drug users, and gays with AIDS, questions relating to sexual preference in many places were tantamount to admitting illegal or illicit acts.

But by what other means could screening of possibly contaminated blood be accomplished? The agent or agents that cause AIDS are unknown, so looking at blood through a microscope was completely useless. The CDC brought up the possibility of surrogate testing for AIDS.

Surrogate Testing and Hepatitis

In medicine, a surrogate marker or test is sometimes done to define, for example, at least a large percentage of people whose medical or blood history would mark them as at risk for another condition. For AIDS, one surrogate test was detection of hepatitis B, since the same life-style factors, such as an active sex life, predisposed gay men to both hepatitis B and AIDS. CDC workers had shown that two laboratory blood tests would detect more than 90 percent of persons with AIDS.

But many objections to surrogate testing were raised at the CDC blood meeting. It would cost $5 to $10 million annually to perform these tests, some blood bankers charged. In the case of those who were refused because of a positive surrogate test, what would they be told? That they were at risk of contracting AIDS? And, if blood were first drawn and then tested, what would one do with the blood that had been drawn and found positive? To throw it away could add another $15 million to the country's blood bill each year.

Enlow's suggestion that "both commercial and volunteer

blood centers implement a surrogate blood test, such as the measurement of antibody to hepatitis core antigen, for each unit of blood collected" was met with silence by meeting participants.

Dr. Clyde McAuley, medical director of Alpha Therapeutics Corporation, a major owner of plasmapheresis centers, announced that company's policy—and one that would be followed in ensuing months by other such collection centers: "We are excluding homosexuals, drug addicts, and Haitians from selling their plasma, because, frankly, we don't have anything else to offer at this time." How gay men or drug addicts—in the absence of extreme or obvious behavior—would be identified was not outlined.

Enlow's suggestion of testing for an antibody to hepatitis-B antigen in blood after it was drawn, and before it was used, was based on the incidence of that liver infection in the groups that had come down with AIDS. Also, there was growing certainty that if an infectious agent was causing AIDS, its route of transmission and those at risk for it were very similar to the people who get hepatitis B.

Two different viruses cause the two most common kinds of hepatitis. Viral A is spread largely through the fecal-oral route and can be contracted through contaminated food and water. It causes an acute attack of flu-like illness with jaundice—a yellowing of the skin caused by the inability of the inflamed liver to filter and dispose of waste. Once recovered from hepatitis A, the person is free from the virus and cannot pass it to anyone else.

Hepatitis B—with which AIDS appears to share many mechanical similarities—has an incidence in the United States of approximately 800,000 cases, with 200,000 new ones occurring each year. Twenty-five percent of those who contract this viral infection become acutely ill and 10,000 yearly hospital admissions are required, with 1 percent to 2 percent dying. Approximately 30,000 people a year contract hepatitis B from blood transfusions.

The illness is also spread through sexual contact and shared needles, and the incidence in gay men and IV drug users is extremely high. Most recover from this form of hepatitis, but some—about 5 to 10 percent—become carriers. Though recovered from their illness, carriers can pass the virus to others through routes that involve contact with blood and probably other body fluids.

In active illness and the carrier state, antigen to the virus is found on the surface of blood cells. In those who have rid themselves of the hepatitis agent, antibody is found in the blood serum.

By testing blood for the *antigen*, people with active hepatitis B would be identified. By testing for the *antibody*, most who had ever had hepatitis B would be ruled out. The last test would effectively exclude most sexually active homosexual men and drug addicts.

The incidence of hepatitis B in America is of major concern, as there is a direct connection between this illness and cancer of the liver and cirrhosis. According to Marcus Conant, if 90 percent of gay men have acquired the liver disease by the age of thirty-five, within the next ten to twenty years, cancer of the liver will be a serious cause of death in that population.

The Vaccine

At virtually the same time as AIDS became an epidemic, the long-awaited vaccine to prevent hepatitis B in those who had never before contracted it was approved for use by the FDA. During the clinical trials of the vaccine in hospital workers and gay men three to four years before its release, no serious reactions or cases of AIDS had occurred. The vaccine was found to be very effective against hepatitis B. But the demand for the new preventive has been, as one publication described it, "underwhelming."

Possibly a combination of factors—that sera from gay men is used to make the vaccine, and that the series of three shots costs $150—has created this lack of interest in an important preventive. The gay men treated with the vaccine during the clinical tests are reported to have a lower incidence of AIDS than the rest of that population.

Resolution—Not Solution

The blood meeting was not deemed a success when it came to a close. "We've been living with this for almost two years now and are convinced of the magnitude of the problem. I suppose it was unreasonable to communicate to these people our sense of urgency in one day," said a weary CDC investigator.

Says Dr. Menitove of the meeting, which left much unresolved business in its wake, "That meeting was horrible. My feeling is that the CDC people convinced the gay representatives that a surrogate marker test was possible. If they had consulted with us they would have realized that it was impractical to set up on a large-scale basis."

But two days later, the politically charged atmosphere was changed to one of cooperation at a meeting in Washington. "We've spent the past two days talking to gay leaders across the country. We'll defer ourselves voluntarily," announced Drs. Enlow and Voeller.

Letters from gay leaders went to all relevant organizations saying: "Don't give blood until the AIDS agent is found."

Each blood-collection agency handled things in its own way while adhering to the guidelines CDC was able to put together. In New York City each donor was given a questionnaire to fill out in private—after the blood was collected. It asked the donor to read the list of indications and to check the box that specified how the blood was to be used—for "research" or for "transfusion." The list included sexual orientation, drug use, national origins, and those symptoms that so often accompany early AIDS—night sweats, unexplained fevers and unwanted weight loss, lymphadenopathy or marks on the skin indicative of Kaposi's sarcoma.

The results in New York were that 6 percent of previous donors were "no show"; 5 percent were excluded on the basis of their medical history; and 3 percent excluded themselves. Of this last group, 65 percent were males.

In an already tight situation (we are not exuberant blood donors in America), the exclusionary practice will result in an additional 14 percent shortfall, if other parts of the country follow New York's results.

Concern over the volume of blood donation was serious, but it was minor compared to the panic in the public when word that AIDS might be spread by routine blood transfusions hit the media.

Soon after the CDC blood meeting, there were two more low-risk, presumably AIDS deaths, though neither was traceable to a specific donor. One was a man who had had transfusions following heart surgery in January 1981. In March of that year, he developed "bizarre neurological disorders" that cleared up. The next month he became ill with pneumocystis and died. His T-cell ratio was very low and no link with an AIDS patient could be found in tracing the donors. But one donor was identified who was on a methadone program to control heroin addiction. This man had a close friend, with whom he may have shared needles, who had recently died of AIDS.

A woman who had died of AIDS had received transfusions during a hysterectomy. Afterward she developed weight loss, fevers, lymphadenopathy and, finally, PCP from which she died. One of the donors of the blood she had received had had many sexually transmitted diseases, had some Haitian friends, and had used amyl nitrite. "None of which," according to Dr. Evatt, "put him in a high-risk category."

In March 1983 the CDC's *MMWR* reported the recommendations regarding blood donations—the self-exclusionary procedures that more or less had been agreed on at the January meeting. Also in the article were the reports of these transfusion-related cases and the suggestion that "physicians should adhere strictly to medical indications for transfusions, and autologous transfusions are suggested." (In autologous transfusions, the patient's own blood—donated previously and stored—is used.)

Although AIDS in about thirty women had been reported earlier, all were in some fashion out of the mainstream—IV drug users, Haitians, the consorts of junkies—and thus disconnected from the general population in the public mind. But these two new cases, as well as the San Francisco baby, were a different story. Now it was "regular" people who were dying and the whole country's blood supply was put in question.

Although the media has been indicted by many for promulgating a "blood scare," and some less responsible publications certainly blew the report out of reasonable bounds, the bare facts, once made public, raised legitimate fears.

Hard data were sketchy: an unknown agent was causing a virtually untreatable, usually fatal disease. The suspected routes of transmission were thought to be much like those of hepatitis B, but that was also speculation. Moreover, there were more than three-quarters of a million cases of the liver disease in the country.

CDC's news that surgical patients receiving routine transfusions had contracted and died of AIDS seemed to confirm the vague fears of those who had been reading about this illness. Many people picked up on the CDC's suggestion that autologous transfusions be planned for when elective surgery was to be performed.

"I've had several requests for autotransfusions," said Dr. Louis Aledort of Mt. Sinai Hospital in New York. "We try to accommodate people, but the blood system can't handle too many of these requests." Physicians in all cities affected by AIDS—and many with no cases—were fielding similar requests; few blood facilities were willing or able to comply.

Another form of transfusions is called "directed," in which the blood donated is for a specific member of the family or friends. Contrary to general understanding, the blood one donates in response to the illness of a specific person usually goes into the blood bank to replace what has been used. It does not go to that person except in unusual circumstances.

In June 1983, after the blood stories had come out, the director of the Red Cross in Atlanta said that as many as four people a day were calling to set up directed donations. These requests were refused, as are most such by other institutions. Commenting on this, Dr. Bove said that routing large numbers of blood units to directed recipients "would produce such an administrative and operational mess that we'd be concerned people would get the wrong type of blood more often than they do now." (Sickness and death can be caused by mismatched blood types being transfused incorrectly.)

Across the country, blood donations fell sharply. Though no suggestion of contracting AIDS from *donating* blood had been made anywhere, the association between blood and needles and AIDS was clearly entrenched in many people's minds.

Hospital reservations for elective surgery were canceled, and some physicians reported that patients needing surgery— and hemophiliacs requiring Factor VIII—were shying away from these important medical treatments.

A community in suburban Long Island tried to set up its own, limited-membership blood bank, and more than one hundred signed up as the organizers went from door to door. Other areas of the country reported similar, but impossible to manage, closed-donation pools.

Separating Phobia from Fact

How likely is one to get AIDS from a transfusion? "It's a hell of a mess," said Dr. Selma Dritz in San Francisco. "I get calls from doctors every day about the risk of blood transfusions. I don't know what to tell them. I can't tell them what the risk is or even if there is a risk."

Bruce Evatt is cautious, but feels there is some small risk. "Of the AIDS patients in no known risk group, about one of four have had blood transfusions in the two to three years prior to the illness. That's a substantial number. To me, it certainly suggests that blood is a vehicle for transmission of AIDS."

But if a transfusion has the element of Russian roulette, there are few bullets in the gun. "In terms of risk to the general population, the risk is very small. The few dozen cases over the course of three years came out of a pool of three million people who have blood transfusions every year," adds Evatt.

The transfusion connection did not go unnoticed in Europe and in France. The Pasteur Institute, in the process of manufacturing another type of hepatitis vaccine, is suing a

Paris paper for creating a scare over the American-bought serum used in that product. "Pasteur Institute Suffers from Gay Cancer," said the headline.

But Dr. Aledort thinks settling the transfusion matter is possible. "One can track blood transfusions. Every time a patient gets AIDS it should be recorded whether they gave blood in the last year and who got it; then find out if that person eventually came down with the disease." But "eventually" means years down the road, given AIDS's probable incubation time.

News of the illness being caused by transfusions and other blood products pushed the epidemic into a new, more publicly visible arena. What had vaguely been perceived as a disease affecting "those others" suddenly became a threat to "normal" people. Only three people officially had been reported as "maybe" having taken in the unknown agent through transfusions, but that was enough to taint the nation's blood supply, in the minds of many Americans. And whenever new figures were released listing those afflicted by AIDS, there was always a small percentage who fell into the "no known risk category." If these people weren't gays or Haitians or drug addicts or hemophiliacs, then who were they? the public wanted to know.

So did the scientists involved in AIDS. Many remained only marginally convinced that the disease was spread through blood. While a good case could be made for that route—the abrasions of anal sex, IV drug use, Factor VIII, perhaps the transfusion cases—everything was still speculative.

Perhaps there was some as-yet-unidentified genetic basis of susceptibility, a common risk factor that had eluded detection. No one wanted to deal with a plot in which some percentage of three million yearly units of blood represented a grave danger to the recipients.

But the three transfusion cases also reinforced the feeling that whatever the agent, it simply was not easy to "catch." The batch of blood that had gone to the baby boy in San Francisco also had been transfused to two others. By winter 1983 Dr. Ammann was to report that a second child transfused from the same batch of blood was experiencing peculiarly severe infections.

While the questions flew back and forth—some scientific, others debated in the media—a new group was being followed quietly, one that in ensuing months would both clarify—and horrify.

8

A Child Dies

Childhood is the kingdom
where nobody dies.
—Edna St. Vincent Millay,
Wine from These Grapes

Before entering the baby's room, Dr. James Oleske puts
on a hospital gown. "This is to protect him, not me,"
he says. In the large crib lies a thin black child who appears
to be about one year old. "He's almost three but he has the
failure to thrive that's typical of these infants."

"Hello, Carlisle," Oleske greets the tiny boy. The child's
mouth jerks at one corner. "It looks like he's trying to smile
at me," says Oleske, "but that's an involuntary movement.
There's something wrong with his neuromuscular control."

"I think his nervous sucking at the bottle is slowing down,"
suggests a young physician. "It's only a few times a minute,
instead of every few seconds."

"Is the CAT scan scheduled?" Oleske asks her. She nods
yes. Hanging over the brief exchange between the doctors is

the fear and expectation of what the scan will show—that AIDS infections have invaded Carlisle's brain.

The baby holds a bottle, but nourishment comes mainly from the lines that are attached to his wasted arms and one foot. The white flecks on his chin aren't dried milk; they are growths of thrush.

Dr. Oleske is possibly the most familiar person in the child's life, most of which has been spent at St. Michael's Hospital in Newark, New Jersey. But when the doctor says good-bye, there is no sign of recognition.

Since 1980, Oleske has been watching babies develop puzzling immune-deficiency diseases—and die from them—at St. Michael's. In this poorest of American cities, St. Michael's Medical Center serves a depressed population.

The parents of many of Oleske's sick children are junkies, some of the fathers and uncles are homosexuals, and AIDS is a diagnosis often made in these adults. Carlisle's mother is a heavy IV drug user who, says Oleske, "is trying to hold down a job and pull herself up. She has come regularly to visit Carlisle; but she is starting to be quite ill herself. She has lost 90 of her 180 pounds." The diagnosis of AIDS is strongly implied.

Carlisle's history is typical of the children Oleske has seen and treated over these years. He was sick from birth. Over his brief life he has failed to gain weight and has suffered from a series of infections, including severe bacterial diarrhea, thrush, and pneumonia. His lymph nodes have gradually become more and more depressed. The present major concern is that an opportunistic infection is responsible for the changes in his coordination and behavior; one of the pathogens has probably entered his brain.

Greeted with initial skepticism by other scientists, Oleske's claim that these children suffer from AIDS is now accepted by most. Although the number of small children in the United States that fall into this category is not large—fewer than one hundred cases—the knowledge that they have contracted the disease has important implications in understanding how the epidemic is spread.

A Reluctant Diagnosis

Without verification that other physicians were seeing children with the AIDS-like disease, Oleske's cases might have remained in a diagnostic limbo for many months. But there were others, across the Hudson River in the Bronx.

Set in a neighborhood in transition—from middle-class Jewish to Hispanic and black—Albert Einstein Medical Center is a prestigious institution. While the centerpiece of St. Michael's is a Catholic chapel that dates back to the early 1800s, at Einstein's glass-and-steel Forchheimer Building a large bust of the great theoretical physicist dominates.

Overlooking this symbol of pure research is another pediatric immunologist, Arye Rubinstein, M.D. He too has babies with AIDS. Most have come from Einstein's sister institution, Montefiore, one expressway exit south, amidst a drug-using population much like Newark's.

While Oleske's office sits in the middle of a clinic where small children play up and down the corridors, Rubinstein's door opens directly onto an enormous laboratory complex. But the patients are the same: they are poor, black or Hispanic, with fractured and unstable family situations.

"It was quite unpleasant, my first encounter with AIDS in children," Dr. Rubinstein says. "It started late in 1980. We saw a six-month-old who had a pneumonia. The biopsy showed a nonspecific pattern called interstitial pneumonia. Then the child went on to develop recurrent sepsis [infections].

"These symptoms didn't fit into any known congenital

immune deficiency. And we did all the laboratory tests to rule out the relatively common immune deficiencies seen in infants. We might have squeezed it into a rare kind of pediatric immune deficiency called Nezelof's syndrome, but we found that the child had a normal thymus and normal production of thymic hormones. The minute those lab results came back, Nezelof's was out."

Having exhausted the possibilities among congenital immune deficiencies, Dr. Rubinstein turned to other possible causes for the infant's immune dysfunction and repeated opportunistic infections. "We thought of congenital infections that might have affected the immune system—EBV, CMV, rubella—but couldn't find evidence for any of them. Then we found out that the mother was in jail. We tested her and found she was immune deficient. So we thought that we were seeing an unusual presentation of a known immune deficiency due to congenital infections."

This complicated diagnosis shows how far Dr. Rubinstein and his colleagues were willing to go to fit the child's immune deficit into a known category. Clearly they were not slapping on a diagnosis of "AIDS" haphazardly. But soon they were compelled to consider this possibility.

"In early 1981 the baby developed lymphadenopathy and we sent a biopsy of the lymph node to the pathologist. He didn't know it was from a child. His interpretation came back 'angioimmunoblastic lymphadenopathy.' This is not a diagnosis you make in children. So we repeated the biopsy. The result was the same: we didn't know what to make of it."

Enlightenment came via the medical grapevine. "The data on AIDS had not yet been published, but about that time we started hearing about the disease at citywide immunology meetings. Fred Siegal said AIDS patients had angioimmunoblastic lymphadenopathy. So we repeated the immune-function tests in the child. The results clearly showed that he had the same abnormalities as the adult AIDS patients. The circle was beginning to close," says Rubinstein.

Before the end of 1981, four more babies with almost identical clinical and laboratory signs had been referred to Einstein. "I made a table of their clinical features. They were overlapping; all the babies had the same symptoms. Then I made a game of it."

Taking one hundred immunology reports from the current patient files, Rubinstein shuffled the five children's reports into the anonymous cards and asked his medical fellows to pick out the children with AIDS by their characteristic immune-deficiency patterns—if they could. "They all picked them blindly from the reports," he says. "At that time no one had one thought about AIDS in children, but I wrote on a child's chart 'Rule out AIDS.' I didn't dare write 'AIDS.' "

A Predicament in Common

Dr. Oleske had found himself in the same spot. "In early 1981 we were getting an increasing number of referrals of children for 'unusual immune deficiency,' " Oleske says. "We tried to squeeze them into some inherited immune-deficiency category, but we had a lot of trouble with that."

Where Rubinstein's quandary was in part solved because of attendance at a meeting, Oleske's began to come clear through his recall for faces. "Our laboratory does the immune workups for both pediatric and adult cases. A man came in for analysis of his immune system and I recognized him as the father of a child who had died the year before from overwhelming progressive pneumocystis. The father was an IV drug abuser. He had a serious weight loss, oral thrush, lymphadenopathy, and a disseminated fungal infection. The immune-system workup showed reversed T-cell ratios. We diagnosed AIDS."

Calling together his assistants, Oleske went over the charts of the suspicious cases he had seen in other infants with the group. "We realized that every one of the children had a risk factor for AIDS in the family. One parent was an IV drug user or the father was bisexual or the parents were Haitian. Sometimes we had to dig; people were reluctant to admit some of these things, but the risk factor was found in every case."

Another child proved to Oleske that he was seeing an acquired immune condition—not one that was inherited. "We saw the disease in one of a pair of identical twins. The sick baby had had symptoms from birth; the other twin has remained healthy for over three years. We were convinced we were seeing AIDS in children."

On the West Coast, any idea of inherited immune deficiency was also being short-circuited as pediatric immunologist Arthur Ammann watched, one after the other, daughters born to a prostitute—each with a different father—sicken and die with the same illnesses being seen by Oleske and Rubinstein. (Only two years later would the mother's AIDS become apparent.)

Physicians in New Jersey felt it was time to alert the CDC. "Dr. Oleske met with us in the fall of 1982," Jim Curran remembers. "I was impressed by two things. First, that he had been able to see that the children's disease pattern resembled that of adults with AIDS in several important ways. And second, that he had realized that there was a family connection. In almost every case either the child was born of Haitian parents or one of the child's parents or a close relative living with the family was an IV drug abuser."

But a problem Curran had with Oleske's cases would also cause problems when the New Jersey physician met with Arye

Rubinstein. "Unfortunately," Curran says, "he realized there was a pattern only after some of the kids had died, so there was not an adequate clinical or laboratory workup to make a diagnosis of AIDS."

CDC people told Oleske that there were also possible cases of the same nature in the Bronx. So Oleske made an appointment with Rubinstein and, taking along the children's charts, he made the trip across the river. Harold Jaffe came up from Atlanta to get information for the CDC.

A Wall of Skepticism

Both Rubinstein and Oleske are devoted to the care of their sick children. Rubinstein speaks of caring for an immune-deficient youngster as "like taking on another member of your family." Oleske cares for children all day and does his necessary paperwork at night. The men were on the threshold of proposing something that the medical world did not want to hear—and they knew it. What was required was a united front, but the chemistry was all wrong.

As different as are the institutions in which each practices, so are the personalities and approaches of these two physicians. Rubinstein has a muscular, compact look and persona. Oleske has been described as "Captain Kangaroo in a white coat." Behind Rubinstein stand all the resources of a major medical center. Oleske's bailiwick is the ten hospitals in New Jersey for which he serves as a circuit-riding clinical immunologist. His laboratory is a facility he has put together at St. Michael's over the past ten years.

Each has an understandably different recollection of their unfortunate meeting and subsequent events. Oleske seems baffled: "I went to Dr. Rubinstein and showed him my data, but he wasn't interested in sharing his patient information. If Arye has objections to my work, why doesn't he call me to talk about them, instead of talking behind my back in a magazine [in an article in *The New Republic*, July 1983].

"All the heads of private foundations in New York read *The New Republic*. When one foundation person who was considering giving me a grant read that other scientists had doubts about my work, he called and asked me, 'What's all this about!' We're a backwater here and we have to scrabble for every dollar we get."

"Dr. Oleske came up here with his data, much of it postmortem information," counters Rubinstein. "You can't make a diagnosis of AIDS postmortem. I asked him to study the mothers, to do complete immune functions on some of the mothers and on some of the live children. But he went on TV and made a big thing of it that was not very favorable for any of us."

The discord between the doctors was only a microcosm of a larger problem. No one group has been identified as being at risk for AIDS without balking, without claiming they were being unfairly singled out. AIDS has connotations that, as many have put it, "make you feel dirty." To the strictly scientific community, each new at-risk inclusion brings into an already confusing picture another element that must be slotted in somewhere.

"Even the CDC didn't believe my data at first," Oleske says, "and I can appreciate their reluctance."

Rubinstein's extreme caution in suggesting he had children with AIDS also went unrewarded. "We kept our cases a secret for some time—though we were being pushed to publish by some at the hospital. We wanted to see follow-ups first." But the first paper he submitted to a medical journal was rejected. In it, he had described "a new immune-deficiency syndrome." "We were very careful with the next one.

We called it 'Interstitial Pneumonia, Hypergammaglobulinemia and Reverse T-4/T-8 Ratios in Children with High Antibody Levels to EBV.' Then we mentioned that some of the
mothers had AIDS—incidentally."

Similarities and Differences

"Initially there was skepticism because some of the mothers
were still healthy, even though their immune functions were
abnormal," says Rubinstein. "That skepticism is disappearing
slowly as the women tend to get opportunistic infections."

The major caveats by the other physicians concerned the
differences in the laboratory and clinical features of the adult
and pediatric cases. Where adults with AIDS become infected
primarily with viruses and parasites such as pneumocystis, the
children get bacterial infections. Also, the immune-function
abnormalities are not always identical to those in the adult
patients.

Neither Dr. Oleske nor Dr. Rubinstein finds this surprising. "This is due to the immaturity of an infant's immune
system," says Rubinstein. "Most adults with AIDS are from
populations with repeated exposures to bacteria, so they have
formed antibodies to bacteria before they are infected with
the AIDS agent." But the baby in the uterus is in a sterile
environment into which only a few potentially infective agents
can gain access. At birth, the infant is immediately exposed
to, and begins making antibodies against, many organisms.
But for many months, the immune system of a baby is relatively deficient. The consequence: "To a small child, the bacterium salmonella is a parasite that takes advantage of defects
in immunity," Rubinstein points out.

"There are no major differences in immune status between the children and adults with AIDS," he concludes. Both
groups have reversed T-lymphocyte ratios, increased amounts

of immunoglobulin G, and decreased T-cell mediated immunity as measured in laboratory tests.

Oleske likens the weight loss in adults to the failure to thrive in small children, which he considers "an analogous syndrome."

Dr. Rubinstein thinks some of the caution has been excessive: "When we sent in our report of the first seven cases of suspected AIDS in children we had to fight with the editor to get him to include one patient because the immunoglobulin G was not elevated and the child had only a severe fungal infection. Since then the baby's IgG has become elevated and he has both an atypical mycobacterium infection and pneumocystis."

Dr. Ammann in San Francisco has also seen several such cases in children and finds the reports of AIDS in infants eminently believable. "What Drs. Oleske and Rubinstein say about these immune abnormalities in babies being different from anything seen before is absolutely true. There never has been an epidemic of immune deficiency among babies before, even in a large city like New York. And a researcher like Dr. Rubinstein doesn't suddenly decide he's going to diagnose a bunch of AIDS among babies without good reason. When people say you can't identify any single infant as having AIDS, I counter by saying that you can't identify a single adult case either. They have to be in context. The context of these babies is AIDS."

The Meaning of AIDS in the Babies

"What is important is not how many cases of AIDS there are in babies, or whether all of Dr. Oleske's or Dr. Rubinstein's cases are authentic AIDS," says Jim Curran. "The importance is that the syndrome really exists in infants."

One of the major assumptions that had to be made to

support Oleske's and Rubinstein's claims was that AIDS is due to an infectious agent. In an editorial that accompanied articles by Rubinstein and Oleske in the May 1983 issue of the *Journal of the American Medical Association*, Anthony Fauci wrote, "The evidence for a transmissible agent being the cause of AIDS is about as strong as it can be, despite the fact that, up to this point, no agent has been identified or isolated."

Such surety also casts serious doubt on the hypothesis that the illness is due to an antigenic overload. Says Rubinstein, "The babies don't have multiple repeated infections. If you accept the kids, you have to chuck out the antigenic-overload theory."

"The babies are a clean slate," Oleske emphasizes. "They aren't born with a lot of background virus infections." Oleske is taking advantage of this situation to attempt to find an initiating event for AIDS. He has begun following two infants who from the time of birth were identified as being at risk because each had an older sibling who died of AIDS. Perhaps a single infection or change in antibody titer will give a clue to the cause of AIDS.

Rubinstein has found that many of his babies have a high level of antibodies to just one virus—EBV. "I think the virus is involved in this syndrome," he says. "We can say that they were infected in utero or immediately after birth. I'm not saying EBV is the causative agent for AIDS, but it may be one of the opportunistic infections that augment processes that lead to dysregulation of the immune system. We studied the lymphocytes from the cord blood of one baby whose older sister has AIDS. We found the newborn's lymphocytes already showed immune abnormalities."

Dr. Curran agrees: "Transmission of AIDS to babies must occur prenatally or at the time of birth when there is lots of blood contact." Prenatal transmission would involve the passage of the AIDS virus across the placenta. Several viruses are known to infect in this way—CMV, EBV, and rubella.

That many mothers appear healthy at the time of birth and some remain so does not bother Margaret Fischl, who has seen several (over twenty by early 1984) similar AIDS illnesses in babies born to Haitian mothers. "We can postulate that the mother has a subclinical case that she got from the father," she suggests. "This is reasonable since several investigators have seen cases in which AIDS was passed by heterosexual activity."

Dr. Ammann, who watched four children die before the mother became ill, says, "To researchers, these carriers are more important than end-stage patients."

"The cases of AIDS in infants showed that you don't need to have an intravenous injection, receive blood, or have direct sexual contact to get this disease," Oleske summarized.

But while the infant cases may have revealed very specific and useful things to the physicians involved, the reports of these cases merely served to fan the public hysteria. The idea that children were contracting AIDS through "casual contact" was the next flap to ensue.

Misinterpretations

In his *JAMA* editorial, Dr. Fauci wrote:

> The finding of AIDS in infants and children who are household contacts of patients with AIDS or persons with risks for AIDS has enormous implications with regard to ultimate transmissibility of this syndrome. First, it is possible that AIDS can be vertically transmitted [in the uterus from mother to fetus]. Perhaps even more important is the possibility that routine close contact, as within a family

household, can spread the disease. If, indeed, the latter is true, then AIDS takes on an entirely new dimension.

Oleske and his colleagues suggested the same possibility in their article. "It seems more plausible to us that the illnesses in these youngsters were related in some way to household exposure and their residence in communities involved in the current epidemic of AIDS."

What these opinions meant to the doctors and what they meant to the general public as translated by the press were quite different. One headline announced, "AIDS Possibly Can Spread by Family Contact."

"My editorial was badly misinterpreted," says Fauci. "It was a perfect example of journalistic craziness. I was addressing myself to the medical audience. I wasn't writing for newspaper reporters. I said, 'Serious attention should be paid to the possibility—the *possibility*—of AIDS being spread this way.' That's all. 'Hey, you out there in the medical community, pay attention to this new finding, let's see what it means.' "

Nevertheless, the news release put out at the same time by the American Medical Association was headlined, "Evidence Suggests Household Contact May Transmit AIDS." The release quoted more from Fauci's article: "If we add to this [incubation time] the possibility that non-sexual, non-blood-borne transmission is possible, the scope of the syndrome may be enormous."

Dr. Oleske also feels his statement was not properly understood. "AIDS is *not* spread by casual contact. I think it is most likely contracted before or at birth, but in a few cases it may be spread immediately after birth. But even then it's only transmitted through prolonged personal physical contact. I'm talking about the kissing and biting that go on between a mother and child. We call this 'inapparent parenteral transmission,' and it is also a way of spreading hepatitis B, which is not an easily contracted infection. But I want to emphasize that AIDS is not spread by casual contact. It is not in the water or the air. The general population is not at risk," Oleske stresses. But he has been quoted in medical publications as saying the AIDS agent may be passed "by other secretions— saliva, semen, urine, and so on."

Rubinstein makes a convincing argument against any household transmission: "Our oldest child with AIDS is now more than five years old, so you can say the disease has been around since about 1978. We have followed the families of these babies and their relatives, and none has gotten AIDS. These people are eating and living together. Where do you find closer contact than that? It's not easy to get."

And Arthur Ammann closes out the proposition when he states, "If this were a terribly infectious agent, instead of my saying there are some dozens of cases in infants and a handful of affected hemophiliacs and those who have gotten transfusions, I'd be talking hundreds."

In addition, a highly infectious agent is not selective, as is AIDS. The 1917–1919 worldwide pandemic of influenza did not respect age, race, or sex when it killed millions.

The Outlook

In the early cases of AIDS in infants, almost all progressed to opportunistic infections quickly and most died. However, there are some notes of hope as babies are identified by risk factors before they develop signs of AIDS, and as treatment begins earlier and becomes more aggressive.

Some optimism concerns infants not yet having been exposed to the potentially opportunistic agents to which adults have been. "The adult AIDS patients not only have AIDS, they have it superimposed on multiple infections that set them up for severe disease," Oleske says. And Ammann cites the capability to keep alive children born with "the usual childhood immune deficiencies," who can be kept well in sterile environments.

This type of congenitally acquired immune lack, however, is *not* caused by an infective agent. The key questions that need answers are: If freed from all infections—i.e., placed in a sterile "bubble"—would these children go on to some as yet unsuspected degenerative condition caused by the virus? Is the presence of the virus alone enough eventually to cause death—or does it simply set one up for infection? No answers to these questions are known.

Dr. Ammann thinks that "restoring the immune system wouldn't cure the disease unless all the infectious agents could be removed." This would include, of course, the suspected AIDS agent.

Reports from England and from Allan Goldstein in Washington, D.C., suggest that children with congenital immune deficiencies are being greatly helped by injections of thymosin, a hormone produced by the thymus gland. This has also been tried on a few adult AIDS patients with marginal success to date. But the thymus gland may play a more important role in the immune status of the very young.

Dr. Rubinstein is also using thymosin, but it is just one of a battery of substances and techniques that his group is working with in an "additive" fashion. "In the test tube we can now see an almost total correction of the deficiency. By using these agents together we can correct in vitro. If you can do this in the patient—not using this one, then that one as is being done now—well, we can see how far we get with plasmapheresis [removing circulating immune complexes], how far we get with gamma globulin, step by step seeing how far we get with each one until you come to the point that all agents are added together, at the same time . . ." Asked if he thought it would be possible to cure patients before the AIDS agent is found, Rubinstein said emphatically, "Absolutely!"

Presently, both Rubinstein and Oleske are using IV gamma globulin from healthy persons. (Gamma globulin is the fraction of blood that contains antibodies.) Rubinstein says, "As time progresses we see that it prevents the bacterial infections. We think that recurrent bacterial infections can suppress the immune system, so we hope that by preventing them, we can halt the progression of the disease."

Rubinstein has had a number of babies who come in every other week for the infusions. "We have definitely seen a significant, remarkable improvement in their immune function," he says. "Among the babies not being treated [because they are not brought in on a regular basis] there has been no such improvement. Only one child receiving therapy has developed an opportunistic infection, a CMV pneumonia, and his parents only brought him irregularly for the globulin."

Dr. Oleske also feels the globulin—in combination with supportive care—is benefiting the AIDS babies. "We have about five children whom we have been treating this way, some for more than two years. None has died and we are seeing improvements in their immune status. I don't know if it's the gamma globulin alone, because we're also trying to push as many good calories into these kids as possible. And we monitor and treat infections vigorously."

The doctor is particularly happy about the first child started on this regimen, who is now almost four years old. "His abnormal immune function was verified in studies at the NIH and at Sloan-Kettering. Recently we have seen a return to almost normal in his immune function. He also has had a weight gain and an increase in his developmental milestones. I'm so pleased that I'm optimistic that he is going to make it," Oleske says happily. If this child survives, he will be the first.

But most researchers feel with Ammann that "the hope is in prevention more than reversing the active disease. That means you have to isolate the virus. Even a vaccine might not work on those already infected—and it may be that AIDS is caused by more than one agent."

There is no question that to have any hope of success in treating the multiple, disastrous symptoms of AIDS, one must "not wait for the full-blown syndrome," as Rubinstein puts it. "You have to make your own definition of the prodrome. I can't accept any definition of 'minor' AIDS—I don't think what you see in the babies is minor—I begin treatment before they become too ill. If you wait, you're whipping a dead horse. There's nothing left to treat.

"One of the first children we saw had only prodrome symptoms. He now has an atypical mycobacterium pneumonia and PCP. We should have started treating him when we first suspected AIDS."

Who Cares for Children with AIDS?

There is no "good" way to care for these babies with AIDS. In the hospital—where many spend their short lives—they are isolated from the normal activities of children, from their home setting, and from the play necessary for development. But the children are sick and at risk for contracting disease from virtually any organism in their homes. And most of the afflicted children are from poverty areas, their mothers on drugs or engaged in prostitution, and home conditions are anything but ideal.

"There are exceptions," says Dr. Oleske. "About half our kids are in foster care, including three we are treating regularly. These foster moms are really good people."

Dr. Rubinstein's young patients are in the same situation. "Most of them have foster parents, an aunt or grandmother in some cases. One aunt who became pregnant concerned me; I was afraid she'd send the baby from her home. But she studied up on the situation and asked me a lot of questions about risk and what precautions she should take. Then she kept the little girl. We tested her baby right after birth and she's okay. But," Rubinstein adds darkly, "some of these babies are brought here and we never see another member of the family. They are left, abandoned."

The question of who has the "need to know" about AIDS patients presents "a tremendous moral dilemma," Rubinstein says. "Once you label a child with AIDS—even the AIDS prodrome—he or she is not accepted for preschool or nursery care. Even 'Rule out AIDS' is enough to make lepers of them. I've seen families thrown out of their apartments because their baby has AIDS."

Oleske runs into similar problems when the children have to be considered for placement in foster homes. "One agency we deal with won't accept the children without a guarantee that they're not infectious. Right now we have a healthy baby whose mother heavily abuses drugs and has a possible AIDS prodrome. I'll write the guarantee and—just to be on the safe side—ask that the baby be placed in a home with no younger children around."

The Women

As the infant AIDS cases raised a multitude of new questions, so did the status of the mothers. Most were healthy at the time of birth: many have gone on to AIDS. In addition, all had a risk factor: being Haitian; using, or living with a man who used, IV drugs.

But, in the absence of actual use of IV drugs, did it mean

that consorts of Haitian men and IV users could get AIDS through sexual contact? Though little epidemiology has been carried out in these (and other) non-IV-drug-using women, there are some anecdotal reports on females.

Early in the epidemic, Joyce Wallace carried out a study of prostitutes in the Greenwich Village area of New York. In a random selection of 25 non-drug-using hookers, she found no indication of the presence of AIDS. But in one young woman—who reported about 15,000 contacts during her twenty-four years—she found frank AIDS. Wallace said the woman died of opportunistic infections after a "stormy course." Her risk factor? Evidently not the excessive number of sexual contacts (she worked in a "fancy house" where, Wallace says, "the girls have to do anything they're asked to do"), but her cohabitation with a junkie.

Of seven of this woman's friends, also prostitutes, two had abnormal immune systems, according to Wallace.

With the number of sexual contacts a prostitute has in a year, and particularly in New York with so much AIDS, why has not this group emerged as a risk group? There may be many reasons: femaleness may be protective to some degree against AIDS; bisexual men are unlikely to seek out prostitutes; it may require repeated sexual contact with a man carrying the AIDS agent to acquire the disease.

The wives of Haitians are contracting AIDS in large numbers—one-third of cases in Haiti are women. But American women also are contracting AIDS from their bisexual husbands. "We have more than fifty cases of heterosexuals—mostly women—who say they don't belong to risk groups but whose sex partners do," Harold Jaffe says.

Dr. Craig Metroka at New York Hospital has five bisexual AIDS patients, three with PCP and KS or lymphomas, two with generalized lymphadenopathy syndrome (LAS). Of their wives, only one LAS patient's spouse has a normal immune system; the other women have various early stages of what appears to be AIDS. All except one of the women knew their husbands were bisexual. Blood samples were obtained from these women without their knowing they were being tested for AIDS. They have not been told they may have contracted the disease—another facet of the always complicated medical-legal question of disclosure. Until they become ill—if they do—and come under the care of a physician, their still-secret diagnoses must remain so: unless the husbands decide to tell them the results of the tests.

One of the men with severe AIDS told Metroka: "It's very common to go out with the boys once every few weeks and go to bed with your neighbors." The man is "guilt-ridden," says Metroka, who asked if his wife knew. "He started crying. 'My wife trusts me. She would never suspect me of doing something like this to her,'" the doctor reported his patient said.

"One of my patients said the seediest clubs are the ones for bisexuals, that there's one here that puts gay baths to shame for pure nastiness," Metroka said. "I think the next risk group will be the wives of bisexual men."

The high numbers of females with AIDS among both the Haitians (more than 30 percent) and Africans in Europe (40 percent of Belgian cases) suggest that being a woman does not protect against the disease, but because AIDS has apparently gotten its start in gay men in the general population, there is little interface with women. Among the Haitians and Africans, almost all men, bisexuals included, are married. It is possible that repeated sexual contact with an infected man is necessary for women to acquire AIDS in this fashion; the prostitutes appear to substantiate this.

Dr. Gene Shearer of the National Cancer Institute has

long studied the immune suppressive properties of semen. He raises several interesting questions regarding how women contract AIDS—and why relatively few have to date. Shearer asks if women who have sex with bisexual men often have anogenital sex and might that account for the transfer of the illness. The differences in the chemical properties of the vagina and rectum are significant and may on the one hand, protect against, and on the other, allow the transmission of AIDS in semen.

Also, many diseases have a sex-related affinity. Is being male a special risk factor—while being female protects to some degree?

This situation was clarified in January 1984, when doctors reported that an elderly woman had died of AIDS. Her only risk factor: heterosexual contact with her husband, also in his seventies, a hemophiliac who had apparently contracted AIDS from Factor VIII preparations. There was no suspicion that the couple used intravenous drugs or that the man was bisexual. They had sex once or twice per month, and they did not engage in anal sex. The conclusions were clear: A man with AIDS can pass it to a woman via low-frequency vaginal sex; few women get AIDS because most persons with AIDS are homosexual men; and you don't have to have a history of multiple viral and parasitic infections to get AIDS.

When this book was first written, no case of AIDS in a man had been traced to contact with an infected woman. The illness seemed to be a one-way street—from male to female or male to male. But in the minds of scientists, uncertainty remained. What, after all, could be definitively said about a disease when the causative agent wasn't known?

After almost four years, after thousands of deaths, after the probable infection of thousands of other people as yet unaware they had been exposed, there were no answers. Only speculation, theories, and hopes.

9

Prelude to Phase Two

> For the want of a nail the shoe was lost; for the want
> of a shoe the horse was lost; and for the want of a
> horse the rider was lost; for the want of a rider the
> battle was lost; for the want of the battle the kingdom
> was lost; all for the want of a nail.
> —Benjamin Franklin,
> *Poor Richard's Almanac*

Locked in a Welter of "H's"

In May 1983, the five research reports mentioned earlier that appeared in the journal *Science* suggested that there was a relationship between AIDS and the new retroviral family called HTLV, or human T-cell leukemia virus. Several of the reports came from Dr. Robert Gallo's laboratory, which had originally identified HTLV-I as the cause of some leukemias, and HTLV-II as a probable agent for the rare "hairy cell" leukemia. Since both of these viruses had been isolated from blood samples of AIDS patients, the American reports proposed them as the possible cause of the new disease. The virus described in Luc Montagnier's report in the same issue was identified by the French scientist as an HTL virus, although it was considerably different from others of that family. None of the articles attracted much attention outside the scientific circles involved in AIDS research.

Almost exactly one year later Secretary of Health and Human Services Margaret Heckler called a hurried press conference in Washington. Introduced by then Assistant Secretary Edward Brandt (now Chancellor of the University of Maryland at Baltimore), Heckler, suffering from laryngitis, croaked into a battery of microphones that "the arrow of funds has hit the target." She declared that the cause of AIDS had been identified by Gallo's lab at the National Cancer Institute, and that it was a new variant of HTLV, which was to be called HTLV-III. That L, which originally stood for leukemia, was reassigned to "lymphatrophic" to indicate what the virus was thought to cause, the destruction of the T-4 cell. The Gallo virus was almost identical to the one described earlier by Montagnier.

Secretary Heckler introduced Dr. Gallo, whose group had also devised a culture of the virus that was to be made available to other researchers, and said that a test to detect antibodies for HTLV-III would be available "within six months" to screen blood donations. Heckler also made the claim that a vaccine would be "ready for testing" within two years, a number she later admitted she pulled from thin air.

With the statement about a vaccine, the low-level grumbling among the science reporters present broke into the open as questions about Montagnier's virus were shouted at the secretary and Dr. Gallo. Many had followed the French announcement of a year before and were taken aback that Montagnier's work was being given short shrift. The questions put to those on the stage by more knowledgeable science journalists were unusually antagonistic. If the reporters could be accused of playing hardball, so could those on the podium. In fact, Heckler's conference was announcing discoveries in a not yet published issue of *Science* magazine—an unusual occurrence, and one that set the tone for the controversy that was to add still another acrimonious element into the multi-faceted AIDS muddle. Another reason for the prepublication press conference, Gallo later said, was that Brandt had told Gallo "they had to make an announcement prior to publication . . . because contracts of $30 million were ready to be awarded for screening blood" for hepatitis B as a marker for AIDS.

During her announcement, Heckler introduced the numerous scientists ranked behind her on the small stage. She even introduced Jim Curran of CDC, who wasn't present. It was a disorderly meeting altogether. In response to later questions concerning the content of the press conference, Gallo said he had informed the CDC in January 1984 of his work and had tested their samples. He said subsequently "that some people at CDC went to Larry Altman, who had worked with CDC, and who is still hand in glove with them, and is in a very powerful position at *The New York Times*. Altman preempted Heckler's announcement with something about the LAV (the French virus). But the only thing new . . . was our work."

A few days before the press conference, *New York Times* science writer Lawrence Altman had jumped the gun by reporting basically the same news as Heckler. Altman's article had been cast in a way that implied credit for the discovery went to the CDC and the French, who by then had decided on the name LAV (lymphadenopathy-associated virus), downplaying Gallo's National Cancer Institute group's virus. The *Times* article was precipitated by one in the British magazine *New Scientist*, reporting on HTLV-III. Gallo's recollection of the events includes an interview with a reporter from England that "the writer said he would hold to use for a radio show in June—but what he did was sell it to the *New Scientist*. Then the press was asking questions. We knew there was going to be some kind of announcement, but we got a call [from Brandt] that it would have to go earlier."

There evidently had been much internecine arm wrestling going on prior to Heckler's announcement. Although both the National Cancer Institute and the Centers for Disease Control fall under the banner of the Department of Health and Human Services, factions of each were being less than cooperative. The Office of Technology Assessment, a congressional watchdog group, published a large report in February 1985, stating that

> CDC had received samples of LAV from the French researchers in May 1983 and again the following month, but had not been able to culture it. In February 1984, CDC again received the virus from the French researchers, and this time CDC was able to culture it. . . . Gallo and his co-workers had their results published in May 1984 and sent CDC their culture later that month. CDC had difficulties growing the cultures in bulk and asked for more culture materials from the PHS [Public Health Service] Science Adviser, who was coordinating the production of the blood test for HTLV-III and arranging for transfer of large amounts of HTLV-III cultures to the commercial companies who would develop the blood test. Subsequently, CDC was given a small, but in its view, insufficient additional amount. At the end of 1984, CDC signed a purchase agreement with NCI for 100 liters of material.

So, "Phase Two" commenced and with it both hope—the identification of an agent thought to be responsible for AIDS—and hindrance—the increasingly messy scientific/social/political realities that have plagued the disease and that have grown in tandem with it. The H's prevailed—homosexual, hemophiliac, Haitian, heroin, hookers, heterosexual, "Horror" (the Zairian name for AIDS)—and now HTLV-III, as another H—Heckler—defused the public's fear of the growing epidemic as if she'd pulled the plug of a dirty bath. The words the secretary used, "vaccine," "safe blood supply," "cure," and "public health problem number 1," conveyed the impression that a solution was virtually in hand and effectively took the epidemic out of the news. After a rash of "breakthrough" stories generated by Heckler's announcement, news coverage diminished dramatically and remained sketchy for the next twelve months. The fascination of the press and public with homosexual life-styles was almost satiated in any event; Heckler put the lid on to take the heat off the administration. Of the scientific validity behind Heckler's predictions, "It was political nonsense," said Allan Goldstein of George Washington University. Indeed, despite claims of AIDS being a priority, administration rhetoric took the place of needed research and treatment funding as investigators turned their attention to the newly identified virus.

HTLV-III: What It Is and What It Does

From floundering about trying to determine what (if any) agent or agents were responsible for AIDS, scientists suddenly had in hand a specific entity. The virus, and its footprints in the form of antibody against it, could now be pulled out, looked at, manipulated—and traced from one carrier to another. That the agent turned out to be a retrovirus, however, was not good news. Nor was accumulating evidence that AIDS was being transmitted sexually to and from females.

"Retro" refers to viruses having as their genetic material a strand of RNA (most have DNA). The life cycle of a retrovirus includes a step in which the RNA is copied into DNA, where its own genetic blueprint integrates into that of the now infected cells. These then produce carrier cells that churn out more virus. Retroviruses also have an exact identification. The three AIDS viruses identified by Gallo (HTLV-III), Montagnier (LAV or lymphadenopathy-associated virus) and later by Dr. Jay Levy of the University of California at San Francisco (ARV or AIDS-related virus), show structures that are almost identical, indicating that while they are essentially the same, there are some differences.

This narrow divergence is one of the major problems that will have to be overcome if development of a vaccine is to be possible. The critical differences lie in the *env* gene, which determines the characteristics of the virus's protein envelope and which must be "recognized" by a vaccine for the subsequent production of antibodies against it. A single vaccine, one designed for example against Gallo's HTLV-III, might not be effective against the ARV strain. "We have to chop up the virus and make a vaccine against its parts. This has never been done before and no one knows if it will be effective," said Nobel laureate Dr. David Baltimore.

The identification of a probable viral cause did clarify in large part the disruption of the immune system in AIDS, however. The T-4, or helper T-cell, is the orchestrator of the immune system. It is responsible for setting in motion almost all of that system's functions: it induces suppressor and killer T-cells; it directly calls up the production of antibody by B cells; and it oversees and regulates the activities of the growth and differential factors of a host of other lymphoid cells. As

Anthony Fauci said, "If you wanted to pick out one lympho-cyte subset to immobilize to do the most damage to the im-mune system, it would be the T-4 subset," evidently the target of HTLV-III. However, several other cells are also infected and may be serving as reservoirs of the virus. The "scavenger" cells, monocytes and macrophages, are also thought to harbor the virus. In light of this damage, the events that occur during the various stages of AIDS are easier to understand, though not promising for treatment.

Not everyone, however, is convinced that HTLV-III is the only virus involved in AIDS. Many argue that although the frequency with which the virus is found has increased from zero (in stored blood samples from the late 1970s) to more than 80 percent in some high-risk populations as the epidemic has continued, HTLV-III may be either a necessary covirus—with the "co" still undetected or unrecognized as such—or an opportunistic passenger. A few still question even the designation of HTLV-III as a retrovirus because of the presence of persistent unintegrated viral DNA, unusual in retroviral infections.

The Blood Test and Course of AIDS

Identification of an agent was accompanied by a method for testing blood to see if it contains antibody against HTLV-III, the ELISA (enzyme-linked immunosorbent assay). Designed primarily to prevent infected blood from being added to the U.S. transfusion pool, the test also gave researchers a point of departure to begin to evaluate the meaning of finding an-tibody or virus in blood. In most infections, the identification of antibodies means that the body has mounted a defense against the invading pathogen and can deal with it successfully. Unfortunately, this may not always be the case in AIDS, and in a proportion of "positive" persons, the presence of antibody does not prevent viral replication from taking place.

Dr. Robert Redfield, head of infectious disease for the Army at Walter Reed Hospital in Washington, describes the stages of HTLV-III disease after antibody is found in blood samples thus: "We look at healthy, positive-tested individuals—and if we find that there's no anergy, no candidiasis, no adenopathy, we call them healthy." The condition of the one tested seems to depend largely on the titer, or measure, of virus in the blood. Gallo characterizes it thus: "If someone has a titer of less than 50, you'd say maybe that was just exposure to some viral fragments and proteins—you know, you put your finger in your mouth or something. That isn't the virus, and they're not infected. They just have protein from dead virus." With a titer of below 100, one can probably assume the individual hasn't got growing virus and isn't able to infect others. "Exposure doesn't mean infection, and infection doesn't mean disease. Infection is when the virus has gotten into the appropriate cell and is able to replicate itself. Even that may be transient because your immune mechanisms may be able to handle a low dose." If the titer is above 100, "that's when you see AIDS." The person is very likely to have replicating virus at that point and is infective—regardless of whether or not there are any symptoms of the illness.

Does everyone *infected* go on to develop some T-cell deficiency? "We don't know that," comments Redfield. "Infected" doesn't mean AIDS, as defined by the CDC. It does, however, appear to signify that the virus can be transmitted. Many think that it's persons in the very early phases of infection who are the most contagious. Although Curran has given "permission" to kiss, Gallo, Redfield, and many others think this unwise, as live virus has infrequently been found in saliva. It may come from bleeding gums and not be generally present in saliva; this is still unclear.

Many thousands of people are going to be found to have low or marginal titers of antibody as blood samples show exposure to the virus. But the results of the test may not be true. Manufacturers claim a very high degree of accuracy (about 93 percent) in evaluating the presence of antibody, but with around six million annual blood donations, and another six million units bought, approximately 84,000 persons will show *false positives* by the ELISA test being used. On repeat ELISA testing, approximately 68 to 89 percent of these false positives will show positive again—falsely. This has the potential for creating emotional, social, and financial problems of great magnitude. Eventually, of course, the follow-up of a positive HTLV-III antibody test will have to be sent to one of the research laboratories with state-of-the-art techniques such as the Western blot test for more definitive confirmation. Without this, and in the absence of any degree of illness, particularly for those outside of a so-called high-risk group (which now has to include sexually active heterosexuals), a positive result should be suspect. A number of persons without AIDS, but who suffer from either lupus or rheumatoid arthritis, also demonstrate a positive response to the ELISA test.

There also are going to be false negatives: the ELISA test does *not* detect the presence of antigen, or the virus itself, which can be present without antibody. Dr. James Goedert of the National Cancer Institute cautions that there are probably antibody-negative persons who are carriers. Therefore, some AIDS-infected blood will continue to find its way into the national blood supply. Another concern is the potential fall-off in blood donations because, as a lengthy article in the *New England Journal of Medicine* in May 1985 suggested,

"As donors become better informed about the likelihood of a reactive test, they may begin to view a donation as a major risk to their well-being"—meaning their peace of mind.

There are several other possible causes for false-positive tests, though neither has as yet been proved. One is a report from Germany that suggests that those with a specific genetic marker (DR4), which is included in the manufacture of the test material, may consistently show positive because of a cross-reaction.

The anticipated uncertainty of test results was confirmed as soon as large-scale testing began in the summer of 1985. A study published in *JAMA* in mid-June reported that an "unacceptably high false-positive rate" was resulting from the ELISA, and that the Western blot was necessary to ascertain more accurate readings. There were also a number of false-negative test results and the blood of four patients with AIDS in the study group failed to show antibody by any test methods used.

The Pros and Cons of the Blood Test

At present, the only "pro" for testing donations is to screen some AIDS-infected blood from the national supply, thus reducing present widespread public fear of transfusions. Even this goal may backfire, if persons concerned that they may have contracted the illness donate for the purpose of having their blood tested. In any event, given the ever-lengthening latency time of AIDS—proved to be $5\frac{1}{2}$ years and possibly as long as 8 to 10 years in some cases—transfusion cases currently in the pipeline will continue to surface for years.

The "major risk" described by the *NEJM* article includes the actions recommended by the Public Health Service following a positive blood test. Persons testing positive are to be questioned regarding their sexual habits and contacts, each of whom "might" also be tested for antibody—which in turn will also result in some false positives. The substantial social and emotional damage done to those with true *or* false positives includes possible discrimination, loss of insurance, loss of employment, and, particularly in the case of homosexuals, fear that their names will go on "a list" of those against whom sanctions of various kinds are feared as panic produces political pressures. The financial burden of positive tests is also an important factor on the "con" side. Additional laboratory studies and physical examinations will be needed, and who is to pay? The unsuspecting blood donor? His or her insurance carrier? The federal government? The United States holds the patent on the blood-test kit, which will produce substantial revenues. The suggestion has been made that this money be used to support the costs resulting from positive tests, for clinical care and for public education.

Another serious problem for those testing positive is: What next? Who is to inform a donor that he or she likely has contracted the deadly disease? Sheldon Landesman says that in New York State, at least, blood-bank personnel will be trained to talk to people. Without question, however, those testing positive will require considerable counseling, perhaps medical and psychological help. There is no provision made for this as yet by the federal government.

Assuming a "positive" is confirmed, what steps can an individual take? An English physician at the International Conference on AIDS in Atlanta in the spring of 1985 said, "To whom are we likely to transmit AIDS sexually? To a prostitute with whom we have sexual intercourse on a single occasion; or to the woman we have been made one with by God. . . . Any woman in this audience today, or any woman in the world, infected by a blood transfusion . . . who will she infect? Her husband and, in passing, her child." The physician went on to describe AIDS as "a very odd venereal disease because the greatest risk factor for heterosexual people is not promiscuity . . . it is sexual intercourse between husband and wife." His meaning was abundantly clear: if you're confirmed positive, avoid intimate contact with others. There is no conflicting opinion about this among doctors. In any event, the "promiscuity" factor initially thought necessary to contract AIDS sexually began to fade away in the spring of 1985 following reports from Cleveland physicians who tracked the illness in gay men with few sexual contacts; following reports of African heterosexual AIDS; and following the increasing numbers of women with AIDS in this country.

Civil Liberty Concerns and Safeguards for At-Risk People

The New York State Department of Health's *AIDS Newsletter* suggests the following:

> • Don't go to a blood center just to be tested for HTLV-III antibody. The test, in addition to *not* being diagnostic of having the disease, may not be reliable enough to prevent positive blood from being accepted and thus further endangering the blood supply.
>
> • Don't be tested unless there is a guarantee of confidentiality. Issues of the MMWR [Mortality and Morbidity Weekly Report] have suggested that positive tests be *reportable*, as are positive tests for a number of infectious diseases. This would result in the generation of lists of names that conceivably could be accessed nationally. The MMWR has also suggested that sexual contacts of positive testers be identified and tested.

• Don't be tested unless there is a guaranteed mechanism for counseling and other needed supports in case of a positive result.

Dr. S. Gerald Sandler, Associate Vice-President of Medical Operations for the national Red Cross in Washington, says that each Red Cross donation center has an attending physician who is responsible for informing donors whose tests are positive. They will be told that AIDS is a communicable disease, that "saliva, semen, and blood" should not be shared. Each donation center has an M.D. in charge who will both speak with positive-tested donors and be responsible for maintaining a list of names. These names will be circulated among all centers to be deferred as donors, "in case someone forgets," Sandler says. Maintaining confidentiality is always a problem, and, although the circulating list will not specify the reason for deferral (which also might be for hepatitis, VD, etc.), its mere existence causes concern.

What Next?

What should those who test positive expect? Current estimates of progressing from positive to the next stage are between 5 and 19 percent. The greatest likelihood is that nothing will happen. However, since the natural history of AIDS is yet to be described, it may be many years before one feels safe from developing the disease. On the other hand, a next stage can be the lymphadenopathy syndrome, or ARC—AIDS-related complex—in which T-cells gradually become depleted and the immune status is put in jeopardy. The "B-symptoms," illness typically caused by malfunctions of the B-cells, include sweats, fevers, weight loss, and weakness. Chronically enlarged lymph nodes—lymphadenopathy—in those with no other symptoms may be a successful defense response against viral infection.

With the appearance of infections such as thrush, however, the likelihood is that the person has indeed contracted the disease. Says Redfield: "All patients I've followed for a minimum of a year, most for two, have progressed. They haven't developed AIDS, but a year later they have candidiasis and LAS. The process may take years and years, but it seems to be slowly progressive. There may be factors that accentuate the progression—antigenic stimulation, stimulation from sperm on rectal mucosa, multiple infections, or IV drug products that don't belong in the blood stimulating the immune system, hemophiliac stimulation, or newborn babies still being stimulated from the mother—all these may modify the time course. But once you develop target cell damage, you'll progress. When we talk about treating diabetes or heart disease, we aren't talking about cure. AIDS probably is going to be a chronic condition we can treat," Redfield concludes. By its very nature, a retroviral infection is chronic.

But early or prodromal AIDS has been compared by one researcher to "reading the Bible and getting whatever message you want from it." A research group studying a large number of gay men with AIDS found six long-term partners (of more than a year) of AIDS patients who have remained *negative* to any signs of antibody or virus. Incidental reports suggest that often those living with a partner who develops AIDS may in some way be protected from the disease. This same situation is known to prevail with mononucleosis, where college roommates are less at risk for the illness than is the general school population.

Acute infections much like mononucleosis have recently been reported to often precede seroconversion (change from negative to positive for antibody or virus) to AIDS. Dr. Ronald

Perry of Australia, who has been studying healthy homosexual men for several years, found that many suffered from an acute "flu-like" illness—after which they were found to be antibody positive for AIDS. Changes in white blood cells characteristic of AIDS took place at the same time. A number of hemophiliacs have also been found to have a "glandular fever" episode around the time of seroconversion.

Paul Volboerding says, "Our studies of patients with LAS often elicit a history of an illness now recognized as acute AIDS-virus infection. We hear about it but usually it's been a couple of years earlier." Tony Fauci has had the same experience, "but because they almost invariably have infections such as CMV and EBV, we really aren't sure if we're dealing with a total HTLV-III–related phenomenon or if other infections contribute to it."

Brain Changes

The confusion surrounding the clinical symptoms of AIDS during the first years was understandable. So many infections are present and exerting varied effects on the patients' status that the central nervous system (CNS) and brain manifestations were often overlooked or assigned to various opportunistic infections. As the epidemic has progressed, widespread and specific changes due to lesions in this system are being recognized.

Cells in the brain and T-lymphocytes share some common molecules, and researchers have found that direct infection of several classes of these brain cells—glial cells and neurons—takes place. This indicates infection of the central nervous system and complicates an effective treatment: most drugs cannot cross the natural barrier that protects the CNS from substances in the blood.

B. D. Jordan of Memorial Sloan-Kettering in New York

has said, "What has not been well emphasized are the *early* CNS problems with, first, forgetfulness, then increasing loss of mental abilities. In 235 patients dementia has been far and away the most common diagnosis. This is seen so frequently it far outweighs the number of patients with no such problems." Many doctors cite changes in mood and personality as important clinical symptoms to recognize, though they may be indistinguishable from depression—with difficulty in concentrating, slowdown of thought processes, disinterest in sex, and emotional withdrawal often heralding the onset of AIDS. There also can be problems with language, with memory, and with integrative mental functions.

These subtle, early changes are difficult to ascribe to organic problems, particularly in persons who know they're suffering from a probable fatal disease. The spinal fluid, which ordinarily will show CNS infections, is essentially normal. The electroencephalogram (EEG) is helpful and in many instances is "profusely abnormal," according to Volboerding. He comments: "A remarkable finding in its more flagrant form are the CT scans [that produce images of cross sections of the brain], which more resemble an eighty-year-old brain than one of a thirty-five-year-old."

The AIDS patients in Miami were among the first diagnosed with infections of the brain and Lee Moskowitz, now at Cedars Medical Center in Miami, has done extensive examinations of brain tissues. Of 52 patients, 73 percent had some neuropathologic changes. Patients were from all risk groups, as well as a number with no known risk factors; the percent of brain disorders was comparable in all.

In some patients, this dementing process is due to various infective agents, such as toxoplasmosis, tuberculosis, and CMV; in others, the AIDS virus itself is present in the brain, suggesting to researchers a relationship to another retrovirus, the visna virus, which causes degenerative brain changes in sheep and other animals. Gallo's group has described a "striking amount of homology [similarity] between HTLV-III and visna virus."

Kaposi's Sarcoma Here and There

Robert Biggar's group from the National Cancer Institute went to Zaire to examine men with Kaposi's sarcoma, which is plentiful in Central Africa. They found *no* HTLV-III antibody in the fourteen Kaposi's patients they looked at. But the KS seen by these researchers is the *endemic*, or *classic*, form. Its course is roughly analogous to the KS seen in older American men.

There is also an *aggressive*, or *inflammatory*, form of KS in Africa, similar to that now associated with AIDS here, and which has not been seen previously in this part of the world. This raises a question that, although it isn't new, has been paid little attention by the majority of those investigating AIDS: the possibility that inflammatory Kaposi's may *be* AIDS. This question was posed by George Hensley, professor of pathology at the University of Miami, and chief pathologist at Jackson Memorial, over three years ago. Hensley suspects that Kaposi's in an inflammatory form may underlie all cases of AIDS. Hensley states that the proliferation of blood vessels indicative of the disease has been found in the tissues of almost 100 percent of AIDS patients examined in his laboratory.

Just over 25 percent of KS/AIDS patients had any external lesions, and these were found only in those with the classic form of KS; the inflammatory type doesn't produce them. The inflammatory type of KS apparently behaves as cancers per se do, destroying the tissues in which they are seated, and is found in most body tissues examined microscopically.

The Miami patients continue to be largely of Haitian

nationality, and include numerous women and children. These also are found to have Kaposi's, but only of the inflammatory type: none have the chronic KS seen classically in the United States. If KS were being caused by a loss of immune surveillance as has been offered in explanation of this disease in AIDS patients, one would expect women and children to develop the same form of KS as do male AIDS patients. This hasn't been the case in Florida. Apparently, it is not the case in African AIDS patients, either. Dr. Waclaw Kornaszewski, chief of medicine at the University Hospital in Kinshasa, Zaire, says that of 64 confirmed AIDS patients in his hospital in May 1985, only 8 have Kaposi's, and all are of the inflammatory type. In any event, KS in AIDS is seen primarily in gay men, and the use of poppers, thought earlier to be a causative agent of AIDS, is still suspected to play a role in this uneven distribution of the cancer.

Of all of the problems confronting clinicians and researchers, the mystery of Kaposi's in AIDS is the most puzzling. AIDS patients whose first symptom is KS are less sick and can be more successfully treated than those with opportunistic infections. What this means is unknown. But there is much still unknown about AIDS epidemic in the United States and abroad.

Latency

A major question, as yet unanswered, is how long one may carry the AIDS virus before illness results. The cases of transfusion-caused AIDS, however, can in many instances be precisely tracked. On average, the latency period—from infection to diagnosis (CDC criteria) is approximately 27 to 57 months. Obviously, many people become ill more quickly, and there may be many infected who fail to develop any symptoms, or in whom symptoms may be delayed for several years longer than even the over five years reported. Dr. Redfield thinks latency may extend as long as ten years in some instances.

Call for a Change of Criteria

When the Centers for Disease Control started tracking the spread of the illness to be called AIDS, their diagnosis in the absence of a causative pathogen was made on the presence of two disease conditions: Kaposi's sarcoma in a person younger than sixty years and the appearance of opportunistic infections such as pneumocystis carinii. These criteria remain in place despite the fact that AIDS covers a spectrum of illness from healthy to end stage; the CDC criteria describe only the end stage.

Paul Volboerding defines the problems: one is the need for a surveillance definition, which is what the CDC criteria represent; second, as he says, "Clinically we all appreciate that AIDS is wider than this definition allows." Volboerding describes psychosocial problems as being particularly severe when, despite serious illness, one cannot make a diagnosis of AIDS, as in the case of severe ARC. Without question, the definition needs to be broadened. With so many physicians complaining about the criteria, as viral isolation becomes more readily available, when an individual who has positive antibody titer and who is shown to have the virus, "Before that person gets an opportunistic infection or KS, I think we're going to be calling that patient one with AIDS," says Fauci.

Art Ammann calls for revised criteria for pediatric patients, saying early diagnosis is needed so treatment can be started. Gamma globulin appears to help some children and even to result in improved T-cell ratios. "The CDC criteria," says Ammann, "have plagued clinical physicians and immunologists, as both KS and even OIs can be rare in these children who obviously are suffering from AIDS." He cites three criteria needed to identify AIDS in children: (1.) a positive risk factor such as a blood transfusion from an infected donor or a parent in a high-risk group; (2.) polyclonal hypergammaglobulinemia (overactive production of antibodies) with T-cell immunodeficiency; (3.) either antibody to HTLV or isolation of the virus from blood. As the criteria are now formulated, according to Ammann, it's like having to have Burkitt's lymphoma before one can diagnose infection by the Epstein-Barr virus.

The criteria were based on the first manifestations of AIDS identified in adults, and had pediatric AIDS been seen first, adults well might have to have the gland swelling and interstitial pneumonia common in child cases before a diagnosis of AIDS could be made. Although these conditions do affect adult AIDS patients infrequently—about as often as KS, for instance, affects children—they are not yet accepted as being due to AIDS. In children, says Ammann, "there are significant differences, such as many having *normal* numbers of T-cells and, in some, instead of depressed T-4/T-8 ratios, these are elevated." One twenty-year-old pediatric patient who is still living has negative antibody, although virus has been cultured from his peripheral blood; because he doesn't fulfill the criteria, he is still listed as having an "unknown" disease.

Regardless of these artificial labels, the fact remains that AIDS in any stage must be treated, and herein lies the final "H"—hope. To *cure* AIDS would require three definitive biologic actions: the growth of virus would have to be halted; the virus itself would have to be eliminated from the body; and the immune system would have to be reconstituted. Short of a cure, a search for agents capable of killing the virus and treatments for the cancers and parasitic and opportunistic infections are the most pressing.

10

The Possible and the Actual

A subtle mixture of belief, knowledge, and imagi-
nation builds before us an ever changing picture of
the possible. It is on this image we mold our desires
and fears.
—François Jacob, *The Possible and the Actual*

"Theories pass. The frog remains," states Jean Ros-
tand unequivocally in *Notebooks of a Biologist*. The
AIDS "frog" is the destruction of the T-4 lymphocyte. Around
this given, theories on how the destruction occurs have pro-
liferated over the years of the epidemic. Treatment is unfortunately also still in the theoretical stage, with both new and
old substances being tried against the multistaged destruction
of immunity. The first goal is to block the passage of infection
from cell to cell; the next, to restore immunity.

"Maybe eventually we'll be able to *cure* the infection,"
says Dr. Robert Redfield, "but I'm a skeptic. . . . This is a
chronic retroviral infection and what you want to do is make
it a *permissive* infection, one that isn't transforming [cells].

187

Basically, you want to stop HTLV-III expression." Attempting to contain a chronic viral infection is similar to the thrust of treatment of herpes infections, where the goal is to contain the virus, to prevent it from causing clinical symptoms and from being transmitted to others.

Since our bodies are capable of synthesizing some 10^7 different antibodies, each able to recognize a molecular structure, we should be able to ward off AIDS as we do other viral infections, but the AIDS virus's unique property is that it cripples immunity. If the disease can't be *cured*, how do you keep it from spreading, how do you make it "permissive"?

Redfield thinks we are going to be able to treat AIDS, and that antiviral agents may play a role in preventing the virus from replicating and causing more damage to cells. He believes that the "present 5-to-8-year survival can be stretched to 10 or 20 years." There are two approaches—suppressing the virus and bolstering the depressed immune system—both of which are more complex than they sound, because we have still to learn how the damage is taking place.

The Antivirals

The cascade of events caused by the infection probably starts slowly. In fact, in most people the immune system may allow no more than a low-grade, clinically unimportant infection, and many carrying the virus probably are doing so quite successfully. Donald Abrams has been following 200 homosexual men with LAS in San Francisco for more than 40 months. Of these, 14 have gone on to CDC-criteria AIDS, while the rest have remained stable. Abrams thinks lymphadenopathy clearly represents a successful immune defense against the infection.

Will the virus eventually weaken immunity in those infected so they progress to active disease over the years? No one knows yet. Will another infection such as EBV trigger seroconversion? Again, unknown; but suspect. Obviously, however, this early stage of infection is the ideal starting point at which to block viral replication. Early in infection, antibody production appears to be normal and there is still response to the test doses of substances used to evaluate immunity. In other words, catch it here and AIDS per se could be prevented. "It will be more difficult to develop strategies to inhibit viral expression in cells that already have been infected by the virus," says Tony Fauci.

At present, a number of experimental antiviral agents are being tried. It's important to remember that we have only a few antivirals in our drug arsenal, and that as they block viral replication, they also block normal cell processes: the line between effective and toxic doses is a narrow one. Several of these antivirals were discovered before the identification of a human retroviral infection, and are clinically untried. One is suramin, which was identified in 1979 as an inhibitor of the reverse transcriptase activity, or ability to replicate, of a variety of retroviruses.

The mechanism by which suramin works is unknown; however, both in the test tube and in patients, it appears to prevent further replication of the virus. When the drug is added to cultures containing AIDS-infected cells, it is able to offer what Fauci calls "significant protection of healthy cells in the test tube. It's easy to detect HTLV-III in normal cells before their destruction, and the addition of suramin totally nullifies the ability to detect hybridization," he confirms. In other words, suramin prevents the virus from replicating.

Also important is the apparent ability of suramin-protected cells to mount appropriate immune responses when exposed to antigens. "Cells can be protected," states Fauci. "They know which specific antigens to respond to and do have an immune program in vitro." Clinically, he adds, "we're encouraged. We're going to have to evaluate the results objectively before we're really sure of what we're getting. If we could duplicate the results in the *Lancet* report from Rwanda [suramin treatment of five patients showing considerable improvement in ARC symptoms in four patients and some enhancement of T-cell ratios], anyone here would put patients on it, but we haven't had that experience. However, the drug clearly inhibits the virus from replicating, and that's very important. That's the first step. Suramin is promising. It's safe to say for HTLV-III positives and even in those with disease, we are making progress in treatment."

Redfield also has been using suramin in his patients and finds that it significantly lowers the level of virus. In one patient of his who was constantly viremic before being given the drug, after 29 days on suramin, the virus was "hard to find, and by day 84 it was impossible" to detect. When suramin was discontinued, the virus started to come back.

Neither doctor has seen any serious side effects from suramin, although numerous other clinicians using the drug have cited severe reactions. Fauci is "concerned that an impression of unusual toxicity has been generated in the scientific community." He emphasizes that "the data don't support this view." The most dramatic side effect that accompanies the use of suramin at the NIH Clinical Center is a burning sensation in the skin after the first few doses, which disappears after about the fourth treatment. These doctors have found suramin to have *no* significant effects on the kidneys, which has been mentioned by other clinicians as a major problem. Such discordant results are not unusual in early drug trials in general; more consistent data should be generated about suramin as wider experience is gained.

Redfield still has questions about the long-term effects of the drug: "We may find out that even though we can't isolate the virus from people while they're on suramin therapy, it may actually hurt T-cells. . . . I don't think that will happen, but it might." Says Fauci, "The one thing we really need are some good early controlled studies proving the effect on the virus—instead of using multiple antiviral agents, none of which have been definitively shown to interfere with the viral replication in vivo—so that you can see clearing of the virus."

Virtually the same results seen with suramin are reported by physicians using other antivirals in treatment protocols. Ribavirin, HPA-23, isoprinosine, and other antivirals, all prevent reverse transcriptase activity, or replication, of the virus to some degree; none halts the disease except transitorily, none restores immunity. On the other hand, experience with antivirals has been limited, and it is possible that more clinical knowledge and fine tuning of dosage and time of administration will enhance the effectiveness of these and similar drugs.

In the absence of a dramatic change in knowledge, Redfield thinks, "We're going to spend our time for the next few years trying to treat patients with antivirals like suramin. If we can show objectively that these drugs really stop the virus—and the evidence is that they will—and that the toxicity is tolerable, we'll move back and start treating earlier."

The Immunomodulators

There are a number of chemicals called lymphokines, produced by cells in the immune system, which trigger the activities of other cells. Interferon is a lymphokine; disappointment followed its promise a few years ago of being a "magic bullet" against cancer. It isn't interferon itself that is lacking; it's our knowledge of how to combine it with other such substances to produce the effects nature provides in a healthy body system. Despite enormous gains in recent years of basic knowledge of how the body defends against disease, we know relatively little about the workings of the natural biological substances that protect against cancers and other diseases. It is impossible to observe these substances working together in the body and therefore difficult to know how to best use those we have identified.

One vital immune-system component affected by AIDS is that regulated by the thymus gland. Allan Goldstein at first thought what appeared to be *greater* amounts of thymosin-alpha$_1$ (a hormonelike chemical produced by the thymus gland) in the blood of patients represented the system trying to overcome destruction of thymic-dependent T-cells. Now, however, he and his co-workers have discovered that this alpha thymosin is "a bizarre type," and think its activity may follow the clinical course of AIDS. The administration of thymosin to AIDS patients, while it has done nothing to restore the T-cell ratio, appears to reactivate T-cell growth factor and provide at least some protection against opportunistic infections.

In the University Hospital in Kinshasa, Zaire, using a "rough" thymosin-5 preparation from Poland, Dr. Kornaszewski reports that he had seen a number of profoundly ill AIDS patients return to near-healthy status. Photographs of several of these are astonishing: in one patient a massive herpes ulcer of the scrotum and penis, which had been untreatable for more than a year, healed within several months. In another series, a cachetic (extreme wasting), comatose woman with many AIDS infections gradually recovered and was discharged. Why seemingly dramatic improvement has occurred in these African patients and not in those treated here is a mystery that Goldstein, working with the Polish doctor, hopes to clarify. Unfortunately, funding for thymosin research in AIDS has not been forthcoming.

Among other cells whose functions are inhibited by AIDS

are the phagocytic ("eating") cells, and monocytes—which, along with macrophages, should be able to envelop and destroy invaders. Monocytes also normally produce an array of chemicals that are involved in the regulation of immunity. In AIDS, the monocytes have major functional abnormalities, and some suspect that AIDS virus in its latent stage may be hidden within the macrophages. One of the known deficits that result from abnormal production of lymphokines includes decreased secretion of IL2, a chemical known to be necessary for the maturation of T-cells.

Many clinical trials are utilizing IL2 with transient improvement reported in many measures of immune function, such as T-cells, B-cells, and monocyte activities. This improvement also appears to hold true for treatment with the substance IMREG-I, isolated from normal leukocytes, and azimexone, another natural immunomodulator. Several other of these lymphokines are under study in research labs. The problem still seems to be in putting these agents to work with the others essential to activate a genuine *change* in immunity over the long term. It is telling, and gives reason for some optimism, that at the beginning of AIDS, even the existence of many of these substances was unknown.

Substances That Work Against Parasites
Some of the major infections in AIDS are caused by various parasites, such as those causing PCP and cryptosporidium. Some of these drugs designed to kill parasites appear to exert their action on both the pathogens and the reverse transcriptase activity of the AIDS virus, and for that reason are being tried in AIDS patients. Among them are Fansidar, an antimalarial that appears to be effective against PCP; dapsone (the leprosy drug), also for PCP; and DMFO (an antiprotozoal against African sleeping sickness), given to those with crypto

infections. While unwanted effects have caused some to be taken off these medicines, those who benefit seem to be protected to some degree against recurrences of the infections for which they are being treated.

Fauci expresses the need for "well-controlled studies of viral isolation, before, during and after therapy, which will establish whether one or more of these therapies will be effective." At present, Redfield's idea for the best treatment "would be to find people [those with pre-AIDS symptoms] early, store their bone marrow, and shut the virus off from replicating (with an antiviral such as suramin). When they start to get in trouble, reconstitute them with IL2; if they keep on getting in trouble, then you can do bone-marrow transplants."

11

Differences and Similarities

Nine at the top means:
Isolated through opposition,
One sees one's companion as a pig covered with
dirt,
As a wagon full of devils.
First one draws a bow against him,
Then one lays the bow aside.
He is not a robber; he will woo at the right time.
As one goes, rain falls; then good fortune comes.
—K'uei, *I Ching*

On Defining a Natural History

No one wants to claim AIDS. So fiercely refused is the distinction of being the population, the country, the continent where the disease had its genesis, that even diplomats are involved in containing news of the illness. But AIDS had to start somewhere. Looking backward and around us now, it does seem that AIDS *started*, that it isn't just an old disease exploring new pastures. If AIDS had been confined to a small, sequestered population, to make sense of what we

195

know of the early cases worldwide, this hypothetical group of infected people would have had to travel quickly and widely during the early 1970s. If one believes that AIDS had its genesis in gay men whose habit it is to travel, this thesis might hold. If, however, the hypothetical population is a remote African tribe, it becomes highly unlikely; few ever leave their own locale, much less their country. AIDS seems to have happened all at once.

This has happened before—a seemingly unstoppable plague that threatened to wipe out mankind. The influenza epidemic in the early 1900s and the bubonic plagues of Europe must have appeared as ultimate destructors of human life. AIDS is unique in several ways. One is its rapid worldwide spread by jet-flying travelers. The other is its total destruction of that system necessary to survive any illness—the immune system. It probably was just mathematical odds that caused the T-4 cell to surface as target. But as was said in the Introduction, something caused the combination of factors responsible for AIDS to crystallize, to come together to form a new entity. As we learn more about the appearance of AIDS on different continents at apparently the *same time*, one is drawn to ever more esoteric guesses. Could the speculations of world-class scientist and science fiction writer Sir Fred Hoyle with his co-worker, Chandra Wickramasinghe—that some new infections may come on us from space—have any validity? Do we even need to speculate that widely?

It would be convenient to identify an initiating place, to assign "blame" to "space," since we likely will never know with any certainty the time and place of its genesis. But that would just make us more paranoid, the threat of the ultimate "other." The *spread* of a plague is quite different from its *appearance*. We resist thinking about the sheer novelty of AIDS, wanting rather to assume it has always been around.

But different strains of flu aren't "always around," and we accept that. Perhaps the disease is so dreadful that we can't consider the possibility that such mutations must happen from time to time for illness to appear *de novo*. But such illnesses do appear, and can again.

Over the years since AIDS first appeared, eminently sensible theories have been put forward to explain the disease. Many work—but only when describing a single "risk group" or population: If only gay men were affected, if only blacks or hemophiliacs, if only those living in tropical conditions, and so on. For a while, it seemed that being female might protect against AIDS and that the occasional case in a blood recipient or sex partner was a fluke. But as the disease spreads into the heterosexual population in the West—it has always equally affected African men and women—some aspects become more confusing, while others become clearer. What is now abundantly evident is that AIDS is an illness that one can "catch" from a person who carries the virus, regardless of whether one is male or female. Also clear is that AIDS seems to require a certain as yet unidentified set of cofactors or conditions to "catch."

A major problem with the absolute identification of HTLV-III, LAV, or any other pathogen as the *cause* of AIDS, is that there is as yet no animal model in which the putative agent can be tested to see if it really causes the disease. Chimpanzees injected with AIDS blood develop a mild set of symptoms but, to date, haven't actually become ill with AIDS. African green monkeys carrying Simian AIDS virus without any signs of illness may provide a clue to resistance against AIDS; the monkey and human retroviruses apparently are closely related. Dr. William Haseltine and others at Harvard are hopeful that the rhesus monkey, long the animal model for many human illnesses, will provide the "best hope."

There are indications that being a gay man or African or from the Caribbean area carries a particular, amplified risk. But is this because of *opportunity*—that is, more AIDS in the social groups with which one comes in contact—or particular immune system makeups predicated on race or on sexual orientation or an already overburdened immune system? Or perhaps there are a number of environmental factors, any combination of which can facilitate contracting AIDS. No one is ready to let go the idea that a cofactor is essential to contracting AIDS, but there are too many to choose from. Identical twins receive identical blood transfusions immediately after birth in San Francisco: one contracts AIDS and dies, the other thrives with no indication of infection. A longtime lover dies of AIDS: the surviving partner shows no signs of the disease, doesn't even have antibodies against it. What's the difference? No one knows. Our lack of knowledge of the natural history of AIDS is a serious and significant gap in our understanding; until we close that gap, prevention will be impossible. It is likely that some people have developed immunity already. How do you determine that, when no human experimentation is possible, and no animal model has yet been successfully infected with AIDS? While it is true that research has never moved so fast nor produced so much basic biological information, what appears to be the easiest area of inquiry—what people are or do that puts them at risk—is still a mystery. This confusion has been promulgated both by those being studied and by those doing the studying.

Because AIDS is weighted with social and political implications, because it often involves practices that are either illegal or considered immoral or, at the least, not what one freely discusses with a stranger, those at risk are reluctant to come forward and speak candidly. So there's bound to have been dissembling by persons who have contracted AIDS. On the other side, researchers of the epidemiology of AIDS have been thwarted by their own lack of comprehension of other life-styles, cultures, and mores: they haven't been able to formulate the questions that would solicit the wanted information appropriate to many of the affected groups. The lack of a cadre of trained medical and cultural anthropologists is seen by numerous social scientists and researchers as having created a major deficiency in AIDS epidemiology. Physicians ask questions and assume they are getting answers, but often the questions aren't understood because they aren't framed in an accurate cultural context. Yves Savain complains that some doctors at Jackson Memorial Hospital in Miami are certain they understand Haitians and become irate when the conclusions they draw from patient answers are questioned.

To understand the behaviors of people very different from oneself, it's necessary to think in *other* cultural categories. This can be particularly difficult for those whose training tells them that asking enough questions about enough things will result in revealing answers. While this works in our own culture with persons more or less like ourselves, the realities of other populations simply do not fit this kind of paradigm. Thus, people such as those from the Caribbean or Africa, and even junkies and gay American men, often don't "compute." They hold pieces of the puzzle, though they don't know it, and the epidemiologists haven't yet been able to find a way to say "puzzle" in these other frames of reference.

AIDS itself is no respecter of race or orientation, of national origin, even of sex habits, but because it began in this country as a "gay" disease, homosexuality is often the template against which AIDS is defined. Many in the science community still think of AIDS in terms of gay men and attempt to evaluate it in other populations against this reference point. This doesn't work. The CDC criteria don't work for the same kind of reason.

As nonproductive as it can be to look at AIDS by separating out different "risk groups," there apparently are significant differences in the illness in various populations, differences that will have to be understood before the natural history of the disease comes clear. There also seem to be differences in the genotype of the AIDS virus, particularly in different populations, leading some to think that HTLV-III/LAV is more a cofactor than an initiator of the disease.

From Men to Women to Men

In June 1984 there were 340 women with AIDS in the United States. A year later, the number had risen to over 600 with CDC-defined AIDS. Thus, the same doubling of cases has taken place in women as in the general AIDS population. The majority of female cases have been among women who use IV drugs: included in this group are those whose babies have been born with AIDS. About 15 percent have acquired the disease from sexual contact with either male drug abusers or bisexual partners. The course of AIDS in females is identical to that in men.

There is no proof of the mechanism by which AIDS is acquired sexually by females; however, it is known that semen carries virus, and infection apparently takes place during vaginal intercourse. How transmission of AIDS goes from women to men is even less well understood, but a number of men are thought to have contracted the illness from prostitutes. Since there is a suspicion that HTLV-III/LAV virus is found in saliva, this fluid may be a vehicle for AIDS in some cases. This remains to be shown.

Household Transmission

Household, or "vertical," transmission of AIDS has not been shown to have occurred in the developed world. There is some suspicion that infection may have taken place through nonsexual/nonblood transfer of the virus in depressed areas such as Belle Glade, Florida, Haiti and in Africa (see below); if this is true, however, extremely inadequate sanitation may account for it.

Caribbean Cases

To explain the commencement of AIDS at the same time in the U.S. and Africa and its rapid and wide spread among Caribbean peoples, both here and in their homelands, most researchers now agree that a connection with Africa is probable. The Caribbeans most severely affected at present are those from the island of Haiti, although few of the tropical nations are untouched.

As here, AIDS in the Caribbean has extremely negative political and social implications. For this reason, countries such as Haiti have resisted admitting the presence of AIDS in considerable numbers, although their nationals in the United States comprise roughly 3 percent of all cases. The actual number of AIDS cases in Haiti itself is poorly identified. In fact, the major source of income for Haiti, the tourist trade, has virtually evaporated because of the Haitian population's labeling as a "risk group."

When AIDS first appeared in Haitians in Miami and New York, where there are large concentrations of immigrants, they were added as a national group to the CDC's list of those "at risk." Haitian physicians and spokespersons have objected from the start to this inclusion, stating that only their people are identified by country of origin; other cases from the Caribbean are identified as "Caribbean," those of Hispanic origin as "Hispanic," and so on.

As AIDS has spread into a more general population, the percent represented by Haitians has fallen. In the spring of 1985, an issue of the *MMWR* ran the monthly tally of AIDS cases with Haitian cases included not by name, but in the "other" column; no explanation was given. In a closed meeting during the International Conference on AIDS in Atlanta in April 1985, Haitian physicians and Haitian businessman Yves Savain met with representatives of the CDC and PHS to request that the reason for the removal of the Haitian cases be made public. "You should have taken more care in saying Haitians are a 'risk group' in the first place," Savain said to Drs. Walter Dowdle and Jim Curran. "We're appalled that the CDC has referred to Haitians as if to rats."

A prime concern of the Haitians has been that their children are identified in schools and neighborhoods as "dirty" and thus refuse to admit their national origin even when directly questioned. Haitian requests for assistance from the U.S. government for educational initiatives to help defuse this situation were not met, and "the press" was blamed by the CDC officials for having caused the discriminatory situation.

AIDS is known to exist in virtually all countries in the Caribbean, although Cuba maintains that its nationals have not been affected. This is difficult to believe, as there are many thousands of Cuban troops in Angola, the socialist country that shares its northern border with Zaire.

In Africa

As far as anyone has been able to determine, AIDS was first seen in central Africa at the same time it was seen in New York and California. There has been speculation among researchers that the disease has been in Africa for a long time, but this is unproven. Many physicians with long experience in various African countries insist that they have never seen the same kind of illness in the past. It is possible, however, that in a slightly different form, AIDS may have affected Africans, perhaps primarily children, and could account for what

Dr. Dennis Burkitt (after whom Burkitt's lymphoma is named) recalls in the late 1960s–early 1970s as unusual deaths from diarrhea among African children. Dr. Jan Desmyter of Belgium proposes that AIDS in Africa represents a more advanced stage of the disease with a longer incubation time than seen in the U.S. and European populations.

There are a number of intriguing puzzles related to the presence of AIDS in Africa. In a case-control study of Burkitt's in African children in Uganda in the early 1970s, blood from healthy children six and seven years old was shipped to Europe, where it remained frozen. When recently examined, the blood showed that two-thirds of the children were positive for HTLV-III—but none were ill. Had they been infected as fetuses and developed resistance? Is HTLV-III alone capable of causing AIDS? Is some other marker in their blood cross-reacting with the test for HTLV-III and resulting in false positives? The same questions are raised by the findings of Robert Biggar and others who have examined the blood of Kenyans from all regions of that East African country, and found the highest rate of antibody to HTLV-III—51 percent positive—in the Turkana tribe, a remote, nomadic people with scant contact with other peoples. Though there is much illness among the Turkana—the typical illnesses of Africa—there is no AIDS. There is little AIDS in any part of Kenya. But this is not true as one moves westward across that vast continent.

In Burundi, Rwanda, Uganda, the Central African Republic, the Congo, Zambia, and Tanzania, probably in Angola and the Sudan, there is AIDS. Looking at the map of Africa, one immediately is struck by the proximity of these countries to Zaire (as opposed to Kenya, which lies across Lake Victoria and is buffered by the politically unsettled Uganda). An international meeting on AIDS held in Cairo in the spring of

1985 included a report that 20 percent of Ugandan blood samples were positive. In Zaire, the magnitude of the disease is even greater than in the hard-hit cities of New York and San Francisco. Estimates of persons positive for AIDS-anti-body in Kinshasa, the capital city, are perhaps as high as one person in ten.

A study by Dr. William Blattner's group at the National Cancer Institute, of people living in a remote village in eastern Zaire, showed 12.4 percent to be clearly positive, 12 percent to be weakly positive to HTLV-III; but there was no clinical illness.

Zaire

This huge country, four times the size of Texas, desperately poor and underdeveloped, appears a likely candidate for the genesis of AIDS when one looks at the radiation of the disease on the continent. Given the lack of transportation and the poverty of its people, the spread of the disease in certain areas—and its absence in others—raises many questions. For instance, the results of the Blattner study might mean a number of things. It could be that there is a subtle, as yet un-detected difference between the virus found in that study area and the one ravaging Kinshasa. If, on the other hand, the HTLV-III viruses are identical between the sick and the well, another factor most certainly is needed to initiate the disease.

The CDC has established a small research laboratory in Mama Yemu Hospital, a large, centrally located facility in Kinshasa, where they are studying the prevalence of HTLV-III virus in hospital patients and members of their households. Preliminary reports indicate that living in the same house with one who has contracted AIDS "significantly increases the risk of infection." The percent of antibody-positive members of such households is about 17, including all adults and children.

If AIDS is spread as is thought, only through blood or sexual contact, and since there is as yet no sign that the disease or even presence of the virus is shared by household members in the West, how is one to account for this? There probably are at least two distinct possibilities.

In Zaire, as in much of Central Africa, the introduction of Western medicine has allowed use of medicines and technologies previously unknown. In general, Africans have in the past depended on their traditional healers to devise and dispense an enormous array of barks, leaves, and such both to prevent and to treat illness. Some of these are effective, others not. Much of the effectiveness of these traditional drugs lies in the patients' belief that there is magic involved. Given this belief and the apparent effectiveness of Western medicine, it has not been difficult for a host of charlatans to set themselves up as healers. Virtually any medicine is available in Africa without prescription. The most popular and widely used way of applying these medicines is by hypodermic needle.

In rural Zaire, as well as in the towns and cities, are countless one- or two-room mud shacks displaying rough-painted crosses over their door openings; these are called "Croix Rouges" (red cross). Inside, untrained men dispense inappropriate medications *by IV injection*. There is often a single, unwashed needle used as long as it is sharp enough to penetrate the skin. Injections consist of substances such as Adrenalin, calcium carbonate, and vitamin B. Persons who feel ill, those who want to enhance their sexual potency, even those who think such injections are magical, spend their limited funds in these "Croix Rouges." The consequences are obvious: disease of all kinds is easily and quickly spread through the contaminated needles.

An alternate, or perhaps additional, route of possible AIDS spread is the living conditions of ordinary Africans. Many members of extended families occupy small, dirt-floored, stick-and-mud huts. There are no toilet facilities, no running water, and most people do not have shoes. Children live on the floors of these huts, and such domestic animals as are owned may wander in and out. A common cause of serious infection is a minor cut, usually on the feet, that becomes infected from contact with a host of pathogens. It seems possible that many may contract AIDS through these unsanitary living conditions, while others do so from the "Croix Rouge" practices.

Unfortunately, there is little to no health education in most African countries, and those governments have chosen largely to ignore what in Zaire is called "The Horror"—AIDS. In any event, countries unable to inoculate citizens against common communicable diseases such as measles, polio, and tetanus would appear to have little hope of limiting the spread of AIDS. Even if a vaccine is developed, without massive, worldwide dedication to eradicating AIDS it would offer little hope to central Africa.

The spread of AIDS there is rapid and apparently inexorable. In University Hospital 20 kilometers from Kinshasa, Dr. Waclaw Kornaszewski, for eleven years head of internal medicine there, is admitting four and more AIDS patients each day. Even up-country, 500 kilometers from the city at Vanga, Baptist mission doctor Dan Fountain's two-hundred-bed hospital is beginning to see persons with suspect illness stream in. Adults being treated for TB and malaria seem to be dying in greater than usual numbers. Even though virtually no epidemiology has yet been done, certain differences between African and Western cases stand out: there is little homosexuality in Africa, and AIDS cases there are exactly divided between male and female.

Dr. Nathan Clumeck, of St. Pierre Hospital in Brussels (as the former colonizer of Zaire, Belgium's presence and influence is still strong), describes a wealthy forty-year-old Zaire man who died in 1982 of AIDS contracted from a prostitute who also died of the disease. The man is known to have passed AIDS to four other women, also now dead. "From these cases, it is clear that normal heterosexual contact is involved in the transmission of AIDS," Clumeck has said.

A Role for Monkeys?

People with limited funds or access to protein foods develop the habit of eating whatever is available locally. In the rain forests of central Zaire, monkeys of all types are caught and eaten. Dr. Joe Lusi, a Belgian-trained Zairian orthopedic surgeon and Chef de Médecine of his area, describes this habit as "eight-ton trucks loaded with all kinds of monkeys," monkeys that are bought by the village people for food. With inadequate cooking, any pathogens carried by simians could easily be picked up. The close relationship between the retrovirus thought to cause AIDS, and that known to be carried by green monkeys and to cause simian AIDS, makes it tempting to speculate on that part of Zaire as the possible site of a subtle change in a viral gene, adequate to create a new disease.

A Tropical Connection?

Several NIH researchers have tentatively questioned whether AIDS could have originated as a disease of the tropics, and some hint that there may be another vector besides human that could account for such rapid spread. Biggar at NCI ponders an apparent correlation of AIDS with the wide bands of malaria in certain parts of Africa. Even in the United States, some thought is being given this possibility.

In a profoundly poor neighborhood in Belle Glade, Florida, home to sugar cane and vegetable stoop-laborers, an outbreak of AIDS that makes the incidence even in New York

City look paltry has been identified. With 20,000 inhabitants, Belle Glade in the summer of 1985 had more than 40 cases by June—a rate of 2,000 per million people (to New York City's 369). Though the living conditions are not comparable to those in Africa, the affected area of Belle Glade also is unlike most of the United States—with extreme crowding, lack of sanitary facilities, and deep poverty thought to play a role.

Drs. Mark Whiteside and Caroline MacLeod of the Institute of Tropical Medicine in Miami, who are active in the local state clinic in Belle Glade, are looking for a possible vector aside from the known transmission via sex and exchange of blood. Whiteside suggests that mosquitoes, or another insect—perhaps as primitive as bacteria—might play a role. Many think this is a fruitless search, as at the epicenter of the outbreak area are both an area where prostitution is prevalent and a "shooting gallery," where intravenous drugs are used.

In discussing the Haitian nationals—there are about 7,000 in the Belle Glade area, 17 of whom have AIDS—Yves Savain cites the use of prostitutes as probably central to AIDS both there and in Miami's "Little Haiti." In Belle Glade, says Savain, "Most of the Haitians are single men and say neither white nor black American girls will socialize with them. So, when a prostitute is available [usually supplied by the gang boss], the men will line up—twenty, thirty of them in a line— one after the other. Anything could be transmitted in that way."

The "differences" in AIDS, then, are many. There are populations with both different genetic and cultural realities; there are different living conditions, different common disease entities, and, very likely, different viral isolates that may and may not cause the same magnitude of the same disease. But one aspect of AIDS that is shared worldwide is the overtone of *guilt* assigned to those who have contracted the illness.

12

The Secondary Epidemic:
The Politics of AIDS

If it weren't for the fact that every one of us is slightly
abnormal, there wouldn't be any point in giving each
person a different name.
　　　　　　　　　　—Ugo Betti, *The Fugitive*

T he disease of AIDS seems inseparable from its victims.
Because those who are afflicted are predominantly
members of "fringe" groups, the general population's perception of the disease is skewed by its perception of these groups.
Homosexual men are thought of as people who engage in
unnatural acts; Haitians are suspected of dark and bizarre
voodoo practices; the largely Puerto Rican and black drug
abusers are characterized as "wild-eyed drug fiends." These
are the perpetrators. The infants, transfusion cases, and hemophiliacs are perceived as "innocent victims."

In the frustration that has been a constant companion of
sick and scientist alike, charges of deceit, indifference, and
discrimination, of withheld funds and stolen research findings,
have been muttered and shouted. The atmosphere of mistrust

has created an ugly frame for an uglier disease. Harold Jaffe has said, "If a Martian came down and saw how our scientific process goes on, he would go home depressed."

Perhaps this interweaving of illness and morals in a sexually transmitted disease is unavoidable, but it has not helped either in bearing the sickness or in searching for its cure.

From the beginning—when the epidemic was called "the gay plague"—homosexual men have been the principal targets of the infective agent and of the anger that AIDS has generated. In a social climate in which many citizens feel victimized by uncertain economic and political swings, much free-floating anxiety has been turned into hostility directed toward this group whose sexual orientation has always been perceived as offensive.

Much of this anger springs from a genuine conviction that gay sexual orientation in some way goes against God's rules and regulations. Thomas Paine said, "Belief in a cruel God makes a cruel man," and there has been much cruelty in connection with AIDS.

Much of the controversy on AIDS focuses on money. The unconsidered assumption that any problem can be solved if enough money is applied to it ignores our many failures to solve even more widespread problems—in science and in society. But with an administration committed to cutting back on health and social services, lack of adequate funding probably has interfered with what might have been done. It has also intensified preexisting paranoia: Many gay men seriously believe that AIDS is part of a plot against them, a biologically engineered bomb set loose to reduce their ranks.

Personal feelings, prejudices, paranoia, and anger have skewed an illness into a social question involving civil rights, the health-care system, the government, and the individuals touched by AIDS.

These social and political realities are as much a part of AIDS as is the novel pathogen that causes it. This chapter attempts to explore the bases and the manifestations of what could properly be called the "secondary epidemic"—the politics of AIDS.

The National Health-Care System

"At a time when policymakers and third-party payers are trying to halt the growth in the health care sector, a national threat to the success of cost containment strategies has appeared," reports an editorial in the *Annals of Internal Medicine* written by physicians at UCLA.

The "national threat," of course, is AIDS. The present and projected costs of research and treatment represent an onerous addition to a system already in dire straits.

Regardless of the state of the economy, the health-care costs of the country move along in an inexorable upward spiral at the end of which—without innovative cooperation among all sectors involved—an absolute shambles waits. Estimated to be $322 billion in 1982, health-care costs consumed 10.5 percent of the gross national product. Each year costs inflate an average of 13 percent.

Hundreds of factors affect these costs—some with minor implications; others, such as Medicare/Medicaid, with major ramifications. Currently, 29 percent of all spending for personal health care goes to these programs. Hospital services account for 52 percent, and physicians' services represent 19 percent of all costs.

The aging of the population as well as the proliferation of high-technology techniques and equipment have exacerbated the situation. The defunding of mechanisms designed

to evaluate what is and what is not needed—health planning—
is viewed by many as creating a situation in which cost-effec-
tive planning must be done in a vacuum, by others as a cost-
saving help. For the medically indigent, free care evaporates
as for-profit medical corporations buy out local hospitals released from their Hill-Burton contracts by the passage of time.
(Hill-Burton was a government-sponsored act passed in 1948
which enabled communities to get government assistance in
building local hospitals, in exchange for which each hospital
would provide health care to indigents in the community.)

Even as segments of the population become healthier
through self-designed preventive measures, an increasingly
larger older population and cuts—or below-inflation-level
funding—of WIC (women/infants/children) nutrition and vaccination programs eat into much of the progress being made
in other areas of our overall national health.

Into this already shaky situation come potentially thousands of critically and chronically ill patients with AIDS in all
stages. Given that roughly 10 percent of those infected go on
to develop the full-blown disease, with nearly 15,000 either
dead or dying by the fall of 1985, cases doubling each 9 to 12
months, and at least three times the number suffering from
some AIDS illness, the words of then Assistant Secretary of
Health and Human Services Dr. Edward Brandt are chilling:
"There is no way in the world that the health system of this
country can support additional thousands of chronically sick
people suffering from recurrent infections for which they must
be hospitalized again and again."

Current CDC estimates are that a million Americans have
already been exposed to the virus. A doubling of cases every
year by 1990 could cost the public $5 billion in hospital costs,
exclusive of physicians' fees and elements of care such as
hospice and home nursing visits. Added to these direct costs

are the losses attributable to illness in the still largely gay population early described by Curran as being 100 percent employed, with an average yearly income of $25,000. The loss to the economy when large numbers of productive young people are thrown onto the other side of the ledger has implications far wider than bare figures indicate.

The care of AIDS patients requires a multidiscipline approach, including specialists in oncology and infectious disease as well as in psychiatry, social work, and community work. In San Francisco, with a well-funded and highly regarded AIDS service in SF General Hospital, the cost per patient per day is $829, for an average of 12 hospital days each. In New York, AIDS in-hospital patient days average 23 at about the same daily rate. Overall, the CDC has found that once AIDS has been contracted, 167 days of hospitalization are required. "Often they can't get out of the hospital because they've been evicted from their apartments," says Roger McFarland, former director of the New York City Gay Men's Health Crisis. A recent article in the *New England Journal of Medicine* showed that over half those diagnosed with AIDS in NYC will spend between 30 and 50 percent of their remaining time in the hospital.

A patient in the NIH clinical protocol estimates that the drugs he has already received have cost more than a half-million dollars. Another with relatively mild Kaposi's sarcoma said, "To date, I have medical bills in excess of $11,000 for diagnostic tests *alone*." Art Ammann is fearful that AIDS will further polarize the public's feelings toward the major population at risk as funds are necessarily diverted from other programs and turned toward the research and care necessary for AIDS. Each disease, of course, has its own constituency.

And, while those concerned with AIDS will find such caveats unthinkable, there are many diseases that affect far more people than AIDS where scarce research dollars also must go. Already, a number of non-AIDS projects at the National Institutes of Health have been cut or transferred to AIDS research; NCI has lost considerable amounts destined for cancer centers, cooperative clinical research, and education, while NIAID has had to set aside work on vaccine development for hepatitis and improvement of the pertussis vaccine. FDA personnel have been redirected to work on interleukin-2 from herpes and chicken pox.

Who Pays?

Depending on the financial status of those who become ill (an employed, insured person versus one who is medically indigent) and in part on insurance carriers' policies, there are a number of ways in which patient care is and isn't being managed. In an ad hoc fashion some insurers have deemed AIDS a "preexisting" condition and have refused payment. A man in Los Angeles, after sixteen healthy years of paying into a Kaiser plan, had to sue to force payment of his hospital benefits.

A significant part of the San Francisco police department's demand for "AIDS-protective devices" was based on one officer who contracted the disease and who was refused health benefits. AIDS was said by the department to have been contracted by "immoral acts," not in the line of duty. The demand for protective clothing implied that AIDS could be contracted on duty and treatment costs should therefore be reimbursible via disability benefits.

No insurance carrier is forced to pay for any medication or treatment that is designated "experimental"; this effectively excludes many of the therapies being tried with AIDS patients. There is also a cutoff in payments after which no further funds are supplied. When this point is reached, unless there are friends or family able and willing to assume responsibility for the patient, the former wage earner is thrown on the mercy of charity care.

Some large institutions are able to manage the influx of patients with AIDS. Dr. Friedman-Kien of NYU says, "We take care of patients—regardless. If my patients can't afford care here [the NYU Medical Center] I take them to Bellevue. The food isn't as good but the care is the same. Those with AIDS are treated like any other patients with an infectious disease."

Major institutions like UCLA, UCSF, and Bellevue are able to care for certain large numbers of patients. The Clinical Center at the NIH in Bethesda takes a limited number who fit their clinical research protocol. But these institutions are exceptional. Most hospitals are restricted in their ability to handle their regular flow, plus AIDS patients, in available isolation units.

Many AIDS patients are already on some type of public assistance. For those lately come to that because of extraordinary medical expenses, there are few options. To qualify for supplementary Social Security benefits under Medicare takes about two years, a longer time span than the lives of many with AIDS who need it. Though there have been requests from many quarters to waive this waiting period, the restriction still stands. At Montefiore in the Bronx, Gerald Friedland says, "It's been almost impossible to get these patients [mostly IV drug users] plugged into the social agencies. I don't know anything about doing it, but I spend an enormous amount of my time trying to learn how to work the system."

Medicaid, the state-run system, provides help for people who meet the state requirements. But most states don't recognize AIDS as an official category, since it is a new disease. Even in California, where AIDS was added to the Medicaid eligibility list relatively early, that move did not mean automatic aid. Dr. Robert Bolan cited a case in which the mayor of San Francisco had to intervene for a patient because a "scandalously obstructionist judge" was blocking eligibility. This emphasizes that qualification for aid is at the discretion of local officials, who may not be sympathetic to "queers."

With hospital costs alone running between $70,000 and $150,000 per patient—most of whom will not survive the end-stage conditions requiring long hospitalizations—there are as yet no solutions in sight. A number of options are gradually coming into focus but none offers more than a partial answer.

Chronic Care

The editorial in *Annals of Internal Medicine* stated that "an unrecognized need at present concerns the care of patients who are ill for long periods of time, are unable to care for themselves at home, and have no therapeutic options." This describes the situation in which many with AIDS find themselves. Those with a series of opportunistic infections are in a debilitated condition even after an individual bout with an illness has been controlled. Unable to work, often unwelcome in the home they formerly occupied, where are they to go? In the unlikely event that the federal government decided to undertake the long-term care of these patients, it would take years to set such a plan in motion.

Under the direction of nurse Helen Scheitinger, formerly coordinator of UCSF's Kaposi's sarcoma clinic, funds have been raised to rent and furnish two houses. "Men whose lovers and landlords have literally put them on the streets, yet who are still able to care for themselves, are being provided a home setting in which to live—as long as they are able," Scheitinger says. The men who become acutely ill, however, must be hospitalized.

Thought is being given to the possibility of placing the terminally ill in hospice care. But a number of constraints stand in the way of this plan. Though the government recently has increased the available money for hospice patient care, it is uncertain whether these largely private institutions will accept people with infectious illness. Also, for a patient to qualify for hospice care, the physician must state that life expectancy is less than six months. AIDS is a capricious disease with a still poorly understood natural history, and few doctors would feel comfortable trying to make such predictions. Accepting AIDS patients is also risky for hospices. Once they accept a patient, they are obliged to care for that patient until death, even if the patient survives longer than six months. Even if only a few AIDS patients outlived the six-month prediction, caring for these acutely ill people would bankrupt the hospices.

Alternate suggestions for identifying specific medical centers as AIDS treatment facilities have both positive and negative aspects. Costs would be lower where a facility was geared up for treatment, and care might be expected to be uniformly good. But making it mandatory to leave home and possibly travel to a distant state reminds many people of the Carsville, Louisiana, leprosarium to which patients, wrapped in wet sheets, were forcibly sent thirty years ago.

In many cities the burden of nonhospital care is being managed by private groups, largely gay organizations. One such program, under the auspices of the Shanti Project in San Francisco, has been in place for three years.

New York's GMHC, with over 750 AIDS patients, has reached the limit of its ability to cope given the realities of funding, 65 percent of which has come from the gay community. All across the country, gay groups have geared up to provide services that otherwise would not be available to AIDS patients and their families. (See Appendix for a listing of AIDS-related organizations and hotlines.)

The Federal Government and Research Funding

Uncertainty over the actual status of funding directly and indirectly assigned to AIDS is barely one step behind the confusion of the disease itself. Some say the government has responded with alacrity to "public health problem number 1." But Representative Henry Waxman, Chairman of the Subcommittee on Health and the Environment, accuses the Administration of playing "an elaborate shell game with NIH money, recategorizing and retitling many ongoing research projects as 'AIDS-related' without a significant injection of new money."

The process by which federal health-related funds are allocated is as follows: the President identifies a figure; Congress votes on it; and the Department of Health and Human Services oversees the actual expenditures. The National Institutes of Health receives the greatest part of research funds, from which it gives extramural grants as well as conducts research and some patient care in its own facilities. The CDC falls under the HHS purview.

The results of this process have not been acceptable to gays. In testimony before a congressional hearing on the federal response to AIDS in August 1983, Steven Endan, Executive Director of Gay Rights National Lobby, said, "Since 1981, when AIDS was first identified as an epidemic, the National Institutes of Health, the world's largest medical research organization, has spent only $12 million to date." Endan pointed out that $11.2 billion had been spent by that organization on other medical research during the same time. In other words, 1 percent of the NIH research budget has gone to AIDS research.

Some of the complaints of researchers about funding for AIDS can be ascribed to their anxiety over what they recognized as a deadly illness before it was appreciated as such by a wider medical community. Most early grant proposals having to do with AIDS were turned down. "I was very aware that the refusal was homophobic," says one physician.

But not everyone agrees with this interpretation. Dr. Zolla-Pazner who, with Dr. Michael Marmor, also submitted an early proposal, says, "It was probably turned down because at the time no one understood the seriousness of the epidemic. Ours may have sounded too pedestrian because we wanted to look at supposedly healthy people, at changes we thought needed following [e.g., LAS]." She does not feel the charges of nonresponse by the NIH are valid. "This epidemic came out of nowhere: under the best of circumstances there is a time lag of nine months to a year in getting grants funded. To say we need more money and need it faster, however, is true."

And Dr. Frederick Siegal of Mt. Sinai School of Medicine, who saw some of the earliest AIDS patients, testified before Congress that the slowness of providing AIDS funding was due to something much less sinister than homophobia. Health planners thought they had "pretty much seen the end of infectious diseases as a major scourge of mankind," Siegal said. "Consequently, we have lowered our research priorities in communicable diseases."

Still, the designation of AIDS as "public health problem number 1" has not always been supported by financial and personnel resources, and appears to reflect decisions made at high levels of the federal government.

A report released in February 1985 by the Office of Technology Assessment (a congressional investigative body) stated that "although insufficient and uncertain distribution of resources has not been the sole cause of delays or inadequacies in Public Health Service AIDS research, surveillance, and service provision, it has resulted in at least inadequate planning, increased competitiveness among agencies, inadequate attention to certain areas which are perceived by many to be important (e.g., public education and prevention), and a diversion of attention from other critical health areas."

The report further stated:

> The history of specific funding for AIDS has been marked by continuing tension among the individual PHS agencies, DHHS, and Congress. Individual PHS agencies have consistently asked DHHS to request particular sums from Congress; the Department has consistently submitted requests for amounts smaller than those suggested by the agencies; and Congress typically has appropriated amounts greater than those requested by the Department. Except when prodded by Congress, DHHS has maintained that PHS agencies should be able to conduct research without extra funds, by obtaining money from their other activities.

After the identification of HTLV-III as a probable causative AIDS agent, Brandt sent a memo to Heckler requesting a total supplemental appropriation of $20,076,000 for fiscal 1984, and a budget amendment of $35,809,000 for fiscal 1985. These requests were not forwarded to Congress by Heckler's office. Instead, the Secretary directed Brandt to "use resources currently available to the Public Health Service." In other words, make do with what's there, a contradictory approach to a crisis defined as the government's number-one health priority.

The effects of juggling of in-place funds and the Reagan administration's refusal to request monies allocated by Congress for this emergency have wide and, many feel, ominous implications. For instance, the NCI budget has, in effect, been *cut* both in actual available funds and in the number of personnel by the paucity of the asked-for increase (3.2 percent) when inflation is taken into consideration.

What this means in part is that, to quote from the OTA document,

> NCI will take funds from its research projects grants center, cancer centers, cooperative clinical research, career program development, and clinical education. NCI also foresees significant problems at the end of the current [1985] contract year when it will be unable to fund continuing costs for anticipated subcontracts at the Frederick [Maryland] Cancer Facility begun with funding from the fiscal year 1984 supplemental appropriation. The subcontracts [would] be a key element in vaccine development and it is unlikely that research can be completed in one year.

The National Institute of Allergy and Infectious Diseases (NIAID) is having problems obtaining funding to hire staff to analyze the results of its five-city study of high-risk gay men, and did not receive an adequate appropriation for its needs in 1985–86. In addition, many of the NIAID programs will be scrubbed, including extramural (non-government) studies of the development of new vaccines and antiviral drugs for HTLV-III infection, and those to develop animal model systems for testing vaccines and antiviral drugs; drug trials in patients by outside investigators and many others will be put on hold.

In the summer of 1983 President Reagan signed into law the Public Health Emergency Act, which established a revolving $30 million fund to be used for urgent government response to public health emergencies—such as the Tylenol disaster and AIDS. The American Public Health Association expressed surprise at the President's action, "since the administration has said the legislation is unnecessary. The next question will be the amount of money that is put into the program by the congressional appropriation process [which has to be initiated by the President]." After repeatedly trimming budget requests for AIDS research from the Public Health Service, the Reagan administration in July 1985 increased its request from $85.6 million to $126.3 million. These extra monies were to come from cuts in other federal health programs.

The remarkable lack of AIDS funding is part of the overall Reagan administration's cutbacks in all funding of health- and social-related programs; and many are afraid that continuing budget slashes will further imperil all aspects of AIDS research. A failure to secure funds has driven people like Dr. Ammann to leave their institutions, and has caused patient-treatment studies such as those with thymosin at George Washington University to be severely curtailed.

Some physicians who have received grants feel there is a "funny situation," according to Arye Rubinstein at Einstein. "We're getting the money for our research in significant amounts—finally—but at the same time the parts of the grant that had to do with patient care and follow-ups and screening . . . all these components were cut."

On the other hand, Congress is perceived as moving in "a surprisingly united and direct way," according to Tim Westmoreland, assistant counsel to Senator Henry Waxman's health subcommittee. When the Senate moved to allocate $12 million for AIDS in 1983, said Westmoreland, "It surely was the first time anyone had heard Senator Proxmire speak in favor of spending money in a long, long time." The bill was offered by Representative Silvio Conte of Massachusetts, a Republican who, said a legislative aide, "was furious and felt the administration had misled him about what was being done to deal with the epidemic."

Making decisions about where scarce health funding should go often presents a tragic choice of one disease over another, and the federal government responds in erratic ways. Why is renal dialysis paid for and not kidney transplants? Why are vaccines against polio, measles, mumps—a whole host of communicable diseases—free, while the vaccine for hepatitis B costs $150?

Diseases all have advocacy groups; but during the early days of AIDS, there were few effective voices. The Reagan administration perhaps is not so much anti-gay in this case as it is opposed to funding any programs that deal with health, speculated Jonathan Lieberson in an article in *The New York Review of Books*. However, the White House staff did meet with Reverend Jerry Falwell's people to "decide how to move on their suggestions about dealing with 'a contaminated blood supply,' " says a Washington insider. Considerable chagrin was reportedly felt in the upper echelons of Health and Human Services, which was completely bypassed by this "health" meeting.

The federal response to AIDS has concentrated on basic research into the biology of the disease. Psychological and social factors, the service needs of patients, and public education and prevention have not been considered funding priorities. For instance, for fiscal 1985, the HHS has allocated only $120,000 for public information, down from $200,000 in the previous year. Both amounts seem incredibly puny given the realities of the accelerating spread of this disease. "How do you prevent a sexually transmitted disease?" asks Dr. Brandt. "The only way I know is through education."

As a consequence of the Reagan administration's foot dragging, concludes the OTA report, "the allocation of responsibility between federal, state, and local governments will also have to be determined, and legislation defining the federal responsibility will most likely have to be executed." On the claimed alacrity with which extramural funding of AIDS-related programs is said by officials of HHS to be taking place, the report compared the "usual" length of time for such requests to come to fruition, with those of the "emergency" protocols. They found that 16 months (as opposed to 18 in the normal funding time lag) was still required. None of this, however, has attracted much attention in the press, and the majority of Americans are unaware that "health problem priority number 1" is largely governed by as little attention as the administration can afford to pay it.

A Virus by Any Other Name . . .

Funding realities aren't the only aspect of AIDS to be taking place away from public and press scrutiny. Another issue with more lasting negative implications was occurring in the research community at the same time.

Both because of the time frame (the French published in May 1983 and supplied Gallo's lab with the new virus that fall; Gallo submitted the HTLV-III paper in March 1984) and the almost-identical viral sequences of Montagnier's (LAV) and Gallo's (HTLV-III) discoveries, European scientists began raising the charge of "stolen" virus. Montagnier put the question this way: If the normal or expected variation among different isolates can range from 6 percent to 20 percent, how could two different and distinct isolates vary in genetic sequence by less than 1 percent? Over 100 isolates of the HTLV-III/LAV virus have been identified so far.

In July 1984 a succession of articles in the weekly magazine *Science* had the appearance of the opening serve of a badminton game. On July 6, Montagnier's group wrote, "We recently discovered a new group of human retroviruses that differ from human T-cell leukemia virus (HTLV-I)." Also in the issue were three Montagnier-signed papers (one cosigned by CDC researchers) and one from Rockefeller University in New York, all implicating LAV (lymphadenopathy-associated virus) as at least directly involved in the genesis of AIDS. Another they had identified was called IDAV for "immune-deficiency-associated virus." The following week, another Montagnier LAV paper was published.

On July 27, in the section titled "Research Article," authors from Harvard mentioned AIDS only in passing as they described the possible reasons for differences in the activities of the three HTLV retroviruses.

In the August 24 issue, an article by Jay Levy of San Francisco identified what appears to be one more isolate of the retrovirus, which he named ARV for "AIDS-related virus," though it was found to cross-react with the LAV virus from France.

November brought a paper by Gallo and Samual Broder in the *New England Journal of Medicine* further describing HTLV-III and saying, "In theory, each isolate might have been a different, newly discovered human retrovirus presenting as an opportunistic infection, with no bearing on the pathogenesis of AIDS." In the minds of those more than superficially concerned with the disease, the kinds of claims that were being made for HTLV-III as "the" agent were disturbing. Of even more concern—had it been widely known—would have been the infighting among researchers that preceded these announcements.

The OTA report succinctly illuminated part of this discord, commenting that the "small amount" of HTLV-III given the CDC played a part in that group's "use of the French instead of the NCI virus cultures," and their signing of the

French-authored papers. "This situation might have been avoided and comparisons of the 'LAV' and 'HTLV-III' isolates might have taken place sooner," continued the report, "if PHS had arranged for sharing of the NCI culture materials with CDC with as much attention as PHS has given to transferring bulk quantities of the cultures to the five commercial firms developing blood tests for AIDS under NCI's license." Suggestions have been made that an international body be assembled to select the most legitimate name for the virus.

By the same token, the CDC has refused to share with NCI researchers any of the samples collected from African AIDS patients (see chapter 11).

A Lack of Cooperation

All along the anxiety and pressure connected with studying AIDS has sometimes pushed researchers beyond the bounds of healthy professional competition. The acrimony raised by the withholding of specific information on the HTLV research from other scientists until publication has been duplicated by equally hard feelings among scientists accusing their peers of similar secrecy.

One scientist who presented all of his findings in a September 1981 meeting was advised by others that he should have withheld it until after medical journal publication for fear data would be used without credit. "I said, 'What are you talking about? This is an epidemic!' " the physician replied. But the information was taken and used in an editorial and no credit was ever given, according to the doctor.

"It has to do with human nature. The sadness is that we maybe have missed a lot of collaborative efforts that could have gone through had people been more cooperative," said one physician.

"Funding is so rare and difficult that people are fighting

for their lives and their jobs. New ideas are kept secret. And [one medical journal] has been especially destructive in keeping new ideas from being revealed until it publishes them— and it takes a long time to publish," another physician said. "It's the part of the disease I hate the most. It's very unpleasant to have to deal with. There isn't any camaraderie, or the kind of exchange of information that there should be."

All who have made these remarks have asked not to be identified by name for fear their future funding will be jeopardized. This is in itself an indication of the lack of faith and trust that surrounds AIDS.

Mistrust of and in the Ranks of Researchers
Initially, arguments between the gay community and the government over ethical behavior were about confidentiality of the names of people diagnosed with AIDS. Much of the frustration over AIDS has coalesced into a running battle over who is entitled to know the names of patients.

Historically, and by law, reportable illnesses such as venereal diseases and tuberculosis are turned in to state health departments with the names of patients. These are passed along to the CDC, which is then able to evaluate trends and disease patterns in the country and to initiate interventions when necessary. The numbers generated are included in the weekly *MMWR* and are circulated to medical and health department people. Cautions about various infectious diseases can be taken when rising figures indicate problems. AIDS was not designated a reportable disease until mid-1983, and even then by only a few state health departments. The disease is now reportable in all states.

At a congressional hearing in the summer of 1983, Representative Ted Weiss, Chairman of the Subcommittee on Intergovernmental Relations and Human Resources, raised two areas of concern: one was that the CDC was obstructing the legitimate work of his subcommittee, the other, that the agency was not respecting the confidentiality of AIDS patients.

The nurse Bobbi, an AIDS activist before his death in late 1984, testified at Weiss's hearing that "a CDC person shows up at the foot of the bed of a person just diagnosed with a life-threatening disease and asks the person to admit illegal and illicit acts—drug abuse, sexual activities, and prostitution." (Homosexual activity is illegal in twenty-three states and the District of Columbia.)

Eventually, the CDC became more sensitive in dealing with patients and worked out a system of codes to preclude patients' names appearing on lists identifying them as having AIDS. However, both the blood test and research studies will run into the confidentiality and informed-consent issues again and again, as there are thus far no firm commitments as to who will and will not have access to records. For this reason, many gay groups advise their constituents *not* to participate in any government-controlled activity.

The Touch of the Unknown

"There is nothing that man fears more than the touch of the unknown," writes Nobel prizewinner Elias Canetti in his *Crowds and Power*. "He wants to see what is reaching towards him, to be able to recognize or at least classify it."

AIDS embodies many unknowns—the illness itself and the invisible agent that causes it. Also unknown and suspect are the majority of its victims. This combination has caused confusion and fear in those most closely involved in patient care as well as in the public at large. Some of this has been laid on the doorstep of media coverage, but most can properly be assigned to the very nature of the illness.

Not since polio used to sweep the country summer after summer has such panic accompanied a disease. And AIDS is the more dreadful because of the amorphous target of the agent—the immune system.

AIDS shares with the severe autoimmune diseases the uncanny perception—and fact—that one's own body has turned against and is destroying itself. And no one with end-stage AIDS has survived as long as five years—the time frame required before a cancer patient is considered cured.

With the natural history of AIDS still undefined and new heterosexual populations gradually entering the pool of the ill, the fears that characterized the disease in its early days are still intense. Persons who had come into close contact (not necessarily sexual) with AIDS patients begin to wonder, as it becomes clear that the latency period of the disease extends far beyond earlier estimates. Nowhere has this been more of a problem than among those who, because of their occupations, must come into contact with the sick.

Hospitals and Health Workers

Reports of food trays left in hospital halls, of a plumber refusing to enter the room of an AIDS patient to repair a flooding leak, of minimal nursing care, and of fears among house staffs have been common. But they are not uniform. From one hospital comes a reassuring trend. Says Friedman-Kien: "We made a decision at NYU that I think was good. The patients with AIDS are not isolated except when necessary; they are not treated in separate clinics as lepers; they will not be discriminated against; they're treated with dignity. We have virtually no problems with any staff." But others have reported problems with staff at NYU and Bellevue.

At Montefiore, however, Dr. Friedland's group has to hold frequent information and education meetings to quell resistance in health-care workers. "It's a terrible situation. We have weekly meetings with nurses, doctors, lab workers. The more removed they are from direct care the more frightened they are. For example, the subspecialty people don't want to do examinations or biopsies."

Jon Gold at Sloan-Kettering echoes some of the same concerns. "There are some doctors and nurses who are very frightened about taking care of these patients and try to avoid it. There are those who have refused—on all levels. They simply say they don't want to."

Sometimes a line is drawn, and nursing staff at various institutions have been fired or have quit. This is in sharp contrast to attitudes such as the one expressed by Arthur Ammann, who says, "That's the risk you accept when you go into medicine. In any event, AIDS does not appear to be a highly contagious disease. It appears to require direct contact—sexual or blood—more than just taking care of patients."

Don Abrams, who was at the same institution, reported that "we had to meet with the pathologists because they were reluctant to do autopsies on AIDS patients."

Small community hospitals with an occasional AIDS patient run into even more difficulty, as their staffs are not geared up emotionally or physically to deal with the immune-dysfunction illness. The administrator of one small hospital was quoted as saying, in response to a reporter's inquiry about an AIDS admission, "No, and no, if we had one, I wouldn't tell you."

Margaret Fischl, who spends much time speaking to medical groups, says, "Some older physicians are reluctant to accept AIDS. They think of it as a 'gay' disease, or a 'Haitian' disease, not as a disease entity that affects these groups. It's embarrassing, infuriating. Some simply cannot relate to it; it just isn't what they're likely to see. But others want to get a feel for the disease as quickly as possible and try to tap into someone else's experience so that they can diagnose it and send patients to the right people."

This dichotomy is experienced in every hospital where AIDS is being treated. "From Day One we have had no problems in this unit," says Bijan Safai at Memorial, "because the very basis of this hospital is people who care. That's the nature of Memorial. Of course they're scared, but they ask questions—and we tell them what we know. We developed our AIDS guidelines even before the CDC came out with any."

It appears that where people are prepared to be sensible, they are. Where there is a will to panic, panic will reign. In the months ahead (particularly if AIDS is reported in medical workers), there is bound to be increased fear, but how much of this is felt by the public is in part dependent on the general attitude of hospital workers and their administrations and partly on the way the press handles these cases.

Studies of U.S. health workers known to have experienced accidental exposure to the blood and other fluids of AIDS patients have not, after a year, shown any trace of antibody to HTLV-III, though a British nurse did die after a needle-stick. But many are withholding judgment on this at present because of both latency and some feeling that fluids from terminal patients may be less infective than that of earlier cases. A 1983 CDC report on four health workers with AIDS who had had no exposure to patients indicated they might have been less than candid about their sexual preferences or drug use.

In late summer of 1983, the *Miami Herald* featured an editorial concerning the death by AIDS of a young, married surgeon. "Medical wagons have been drawn into a circle of silence as tight as if hostile scalp-hunters were circling the dead physician's reputation," the newspaper said. "The truth might not be pleasant or tidy, but it cannot possibly be as threatening as the rumors and fears that multiply in a climate of mystery." The editorial was titled, "Tell the Truth."

But the truth about AIDS has a multiplicity of faces, largely due to the connotations of how and what one is and does to contract the illness. A number of health workers have indeed been infected with AIDS and most of these have died. One scare at NYU well describes the problems inherent in assigning the source of the infection. Reports Dr. Metroka: "The husband of a nurse who took care of AIDS patients died of PCP and toxoplasmosis of the central nervous system. She said absolutely that he was neither a homosexual nor an IV drug user. But we checked his hospital records of several years earlier and saw that he had previously admitted both IV drug use and male sexual contacts."

Finding virus in the saliva of well people at risk for AIDS has exacerbated anxiety in some hospital personnel. "I don't want to be alarmist," said Gallo, who found the virus, and who feels it can't be transmitted through casual contact, "certainly not by a peck [kiss] or by [drinking from] a glass."

Dan William, in New York, describes his experience with hospitalized patients as "not as bad as some I've heard. But sometimes a patient will be admitted into a semiprivate room for evaluation because we suspect AIDS and what happens is that the family of the other patient asks that he be transferred to another room. This has been a source of frustration because people are constantly being moved around. I never know where I'll find my patients."

Though the usual precautions for dealing with patients with infectious diseases—"needle and stool precautions"— would appear to be adequate, there still are those too afraid to get near AIDS patients without what Jon Gold calls "unnecessary precautions." "When patients are put in a room that no one enters without wearing masks and gowns, the tendency is for doctors and nurses and aides to go in as little as they can. So these patients are ostracized; it depresses them and it may compromise their care, so we try not to let it happen."

But it does happen, says Dr. Ammann. "AIDS patients are the lepers of today. They're dying under the gaze of only a pair of reluctant eyes peering over a mask."

A man who came across the country to see a former lover who was dying said the experience "shattered" him. "All I could think of—and still do—all the damned time is that he was lying there dying and all he ever saw of another human being was a mask."

The medical personnel "burnout" in hospitals with large populations of AIDS patients is considerable. Dr. Friedland graphically—and wearily—describes his own experience: "The excitement of a new disease entity has completely left me now. I had some patients who seemed to be doing so well and all of a sudden they crashed, and all I have is young people dying. It's been like going to a foreign country [he was in the Peace Corps in Nigeria a number of years ago]: you feel the initial excitement for a while, then the reality hits and you have to contend with that reality. This is a hard one."

A nurse in California who has been working with AIDS for several years had to ask for a transfer. "I got to the point that I wanted to scream or cry or just run away every time I walked into another young, dying man's room. And there were the nightmares. . . ."

An even more subtle problem has been encountered by dermatologist Patrick Hennessey, whose office staff, though careful of potential AIDS-containing material, is not in the least frightened. Describing his excellent relationship with his family, many of whom are in various areas of health care, Hennessey was concerned that the chronically poor health of his sister's two-year-old twins must raise questions: "It's like if the babies are having problems—and I spent much time with them right after they were born—who is going to be the first to ask if it could be related to me?" Fortunately, the children appear to be growing up in good health.

In New York, the union representing prison guards demanded that prisoners with AIDS be isolated and that guards be given protective clothing to wear when dealing with these men. The statement in *JAMA* suggesting that "routine close contact" might possibly spread the disease was cited as a rationale for the union demands.

On the heels of the guards' demands, the New York Funeral Directors' Association gave notice that their members would not embalm those who had died of AIDS until strict guidelines were laid down by the government. There are many stories of unwashed bodies being buried in closed plastic bags doused with embalming fluid, of refusal to open caskets for relatives, and difficulty in the shipment of bodies to other states for burial.

In the wake of what is perceived as discrimination against homosexuals, the Lambda Legal Defense and Education Fund of New York has brought suit against employers who have fired healthy gays because of the AIDS scare, and negotiations are being conducted with many others. Suits are being contemplated against schools that deny the children of AIDS victims admittance and against the Air Force, which denied medical benefits to a soldier on grounds he had contracted the disease because of "misconduct." He subsequently received a medical discharge and full benefits. Several men in other armed services have been medically retired or are on convalescent leave because of having contracted AIDS. There has been relatively little quibbling over this by the various involved branches of the military.

Homophiles and Homophobes

At the rock bottom of most thinking about AIDS—solidly entrenched, whether by groups or individuals, gay or straight— is a powerful opinion vis-à-vis homosexuality.

The general consensus is that because of their numbers, their having first contracted the disease, and the attitudes of the majority of people, responsibility for AIDS rests squarely on the heads of gay men. Regardless of what is eventually discovered about the immune-system breakdown, its origins and modes of transmission, AIDS will likely go down in history as the "Gay Plague."

In the minds of most people, homosexuals are lumped together, with little distinction being made between male and female, "liberal" and "conservative," swingers and old settled couples. Parameters need to be drawn to clarify what is meant by "promiscuous"; terms bandied about in the media such as "fast-lane life-styles," "sexually active," or "monogamous gays" have to be more clearly defined.

Stonewall and Beyond

The drastic changes in homosexual visibility and activity and the resultant changes in life styles—to which much of the spread of AIDS is ascribed—are rooted in social mores. Some of the practices of gay men, about which much has been written and on which much of the "blame" for AIDS has been laid, need to be seen in an overall social context. Also, the deep concern of the gay population regarding their position in "post-AIDS" society bears on the political rhetoric now being expressed.

Good, bad, or indifferent, homosexuality is a fact of human life; personal judgments about it have no place in the context of the disease that is creating such devastation among gay men. Changes over the past fifteen years have altered public perception of homosexuals to some degree; those changes certainly have affected gay perception to a great degree.

Twenty years ago few men chose to reveal publicly that their sexual orientation was to other men. They were "closeted," which meant that they acted and dressed in what is perceived to be a "straight" way and hid their homosexuality from most of the world. In the dawning sexual permissiveness of the 1960s, this began to change. It was brought to a crisis by what Dr. Dan William calls "a warm summer night in June 1969," when police raided the Stonewall, a popular gay disco in New York's Greenwich Village. The raid set off riots that eventuated in a huge parade up Fifth Avenue. Gay men and women marched for their civil rights and came out of the closet en masse, once and for all.

Repressed socially, sexually, and psychically for so long, like the children of the Victorians, the gays let it all loose. While straights became "swingers," lived together unmarried, and even middle-class suburban couples participated in partner swapping and group sex, gay men set about creating their own sexual revolution—which accommodated a range that is marked by as many individual styles and forms of sexual expression as the heterosexual sexual revolution.

Older men who had gained acceptance at work and in social settings changed little in their lives. Most had evolved stable relationships within a coterie of like men and, though perhaps regarded as "probably queer" by others, found it no impediment in their lives. These are men for whom the idea of "swinging" in any context simply was not at all attractive.

But for the young, and for the profoundly closeted, this was the beginning of a mass coming-out. As Marcus Conant puts it, "Overt sexuality is the statement of many gay men." They chose to express formerly forbidden sexual interest in other men partly as an expression of what has come to be called "gay pride."

In 1973, the American Medical Association's Council on Scientific Affairs reported to its members: "The task force of the American Psychiatric Association that addressed homosexuality indicated that it was impossible to differentiate between homosexuals and heterosexuals on the basis of tests for psychological and social functioning." On the basis of that report, the APA voted to declassify homosexuality as an illness and to remove it from its official list of mental disorders.

Life-styles

The general perception of the male homosexual as an effeminate, limp-wristed "faggot" does not fit most gay men. Drag "queens" and transvestites make up a tiny minority in the overall gay population. The "macho" or "leather" image attracts only a small subset of gays. Overtly, the great majority of America's gay men are indistinguishable from "straights."

Most gay men fit into several well-defined categories of relationships. (It should be emphasized, however, that these rubrics do not encompass the subtleties of a wide range of possible life-styles followed by gays.) The 1978 book *Homosexualities: A Study of Diversity Among Men and Women*, by Alan P. Bell and Martin S. Weinberg, lists the following general categories into which most gay men fall:

- *Closed couples* closely resemble heterosexual pairs. They are relatively monogamous, have few

problems regarding their sexual orientation, and do
not participate in a fast-lane life-style.

• *Open couples* maintain a special one-on-one
relationship while keeping up outside social and sexual activities. These men appeared to the authors to
be less comfortable with their identities and relationships than the closed couples.

• *Functionals* are described as being the most
satisfied with being gay and conduct active, free-
wheeling sex lives comparable to "swinging singles"
in the heterosexual world. While these men have
positive self-images, they appear to be more lonely
and anxious than those who have established satis-
fying monogamous relationships. (The same holds
true for many unmarried or uncommitted straight
people.)

• *Dysfunctionals* are those who are dissatisfied
with their sexual orientation both socially and sexually. This group probably represents the 15 percent
of gay men estimated by the AMA as those who
would prefer being heterosexual.

In all cases, life-style is in great part determined by age,
education, and upbringing.

One of the problems encountered by epidemiologists attempting to define the behavioral patterns in the three major
groups at risk for AIDS—gay men, Haitians, and drug abusers—parallels the problems of anthropologists: it is extremely
hard even to ask the right questions without having a solid
understanding of a culture. The word "promiscuous," for example, means one thing to a middle-class heterosexual man
and something else when used in gay parlance. In the same

way, trying to translate the jargon used by IV drug abusers and the cultural mores of Haitians has presented a sizable problem for researchers.

Race also plays a part: in many nonwhite cultures, a man who takes a masculine, penetrative role in sexual acts is not perceived as homosexual—regardless of the gender of his sexual partner. One of the physicians conducting early research on the Haitians discovered that the Creole word he thought meant "homosexual" in fact meant "transvestite," and applies only to those who take a passive role in intercourse. Haitians are more concerned with the *masculinity* of the sex role; Americans tend to be more aware of what appear to be the *morals* of the act.

Differing attitudes toward sex roles are well defined in men's prisons, where more than 55 percent of heterosexual men are known to participate in various sexual practices with one another. In their book *Men Behind Bars*, authors Wayne S. Wooden and Jay Parker report on a middle-security prison in California in which heterosexual men almost always take the active, or penetrative, role—unless they are raped by other inmates. These men either anally penetrated others or had fellatio performed on them. They did not consider themselves homosexual and, when released from prison, returned to their previous preference for women.

Attitude

Writing in the *California Voice*, Dr. Tom Waddell states, "We have probed a particular theme in our lives which we call sexual freedom and have crossed some natural barrier." While Waddell refers to the series of infections to which gay men are subject, it is also perceived that the "natural barrier" is a personal and social one and that AIDS may be a perverse intruder that will call a halt to obsessive preoccupation with sex.

Larry Kramer berates his fellows in a *New York Native* article for their lethargy in failing to organize in a timely manner to combat AIDS: "I'm sick of guys who think that all that being gay means is sex in the first place." Kramer cites this preoccupation as having made for miserable human relationships and a self-destructive mode of behavior for which disease is a logical companion. "I get furious at guys who say, 'Oh, look at what they've done to us!' We've done it to us! I know we've got historical reasons for being oppressed, but everybody's oppressed: women are oppressed, Jews are oppressed, blacks are oppressed, Hispanics are oppressed. And you can lie down and be a carpet or you can fight back. . . . It's ironic that the whole political platform of the gay liberation has been based on sexual revolution and now we find that that's got poison darts in it."

One of the "poison darts" is the kind of relationship that develops out of such a life-style. In Los Angeles's *Advocate,* Carl Maves writes:

> Attitude: it's a word we use daily but never have bothered to define. It's a sickness. Or is it a kindness? It's arrogance. Or is it self-defense? It's something we pick up in dismay and put down in anger. Look, over there, that guy's giving me ATTITUDE! OK for you, asshole, guess what you're getting back? More attitude, of course. And more and more and still more until the attitude multiplies like an image in a hall of mirrors. The image is a ghost, and the hall is a dead-end . . . look! The face in the mirror is: Yours. And mine. Face it, friend, we all give attitude because we all get it and want to get back at those who give it. And they are us.

"Attitude" in this frame of reference is a ghetto term picked up by gays. It is the mask worn to protect against loneliness and uncertainty, the guise in which a man can cruise the bars and baths and not be crushed by being ignored or put down by others. It's the pose that says, "I don't give a damn about you, either." "It's a nasty little weapon," says Maves. "It doesn't cut clean."

This "attitude" and the shallowness of many relationships it produces have made themselves painfully evident since the AIDS crisis began. Where liaisons are based solely on sexual attraction, the mere suggestion of AIDS in one man has resulted in brutal emotional and physical rejection by the other. There are many stories of men returning home from work or the hospital to find their belongings in the street or burned, the house locked against them, telephone calls unanswered. A formerly wealthy West Coast publisher found himself standing in the middle of the street clutching all that remained of his possessions in a small plastic bag. AIDS and his former friends had literally done away with all else he had ever owned.

Many parents have been unable and unwilling to deal with their sick sons: "My father said he couldn't do anything about any of it so I should just leave him alone—disappear," said a man with KS. There have been reports of suicides and deep mental disorders and sheer panic heaped on top of this disease. But there also have been many more instances of care and loyalty. The concept of "brotherhood" has begun to take on new meaning for many homosexuals. The father of a young man with AIDS has said, "You know, when something like this hits *your* family, it's not a 'gay disease,' it's a very serious disease that has struck someone you love."

Gay Support Groups

AIDS well may be the potential seed of a genuine political revolution in America. There has been a drawing together into substantial organizations of those concerned with the illness—patients, physicians, families, and friends. The often used term "gay community" really had scant relevance before the threat of AIDS. Newly formed groups have appeared in most communities affected by the disease, and those in the major areas are providing a multitude of essential human services.

Curled small in the corner of the sofa in his library-like apartment, Mitchell Cutler quietly speaks of his fears and his newfound pride. "For the first time in my life I feel as if I'm contributing something valuable, and it makes me feel good; it makes all of us in the group feel good about ourselves." A dealer in rare art books, Cutler dismisses his esoteric occupation as "hardly a major contribution to society—selling expensive books to rich people." He now spends the majority of his time recruiting, training, and directing the more than fifty volunteers who provide a spectrum of services for those with AIDS. "We walk dogs, deliver prepared meals, take people back and forth to meetings and doctor appointments, clean apartments, help move—whatever needs doing and they can't do for themselves.

"One of the men was just released from the hospital and walks with a walker, so someone goes by and makes him breakfast and leaves his lunch, and someone else goes to make his dinner. And one man who was being transferred from the hospital part of NYU to the co-op care unit, well, when the doctor couldn't absolutely guarantee that he was completely recovered from his pneumocystis, that there were no traces of it left, the poor guy called me late in the evening and said he'd packed and unpacked, and had to pack and move again all in the space of a day. He was exhausted and disappointed. He was so sad; he'd been in the hospital for eight weeks. So I arranged for the men who were going to take care of him in co-op to do the same in his home. The guys put in a lot of work. It's really an extraordinary privilege to work with these people. They are very dedicated and have a lot of real compassion.

"I have another man who picks up someone in Brooklyn every Wednesday evening to take him to the AIDS support group in Manhattan. He waits, then drives him home again. This same Buddy also baby-sits for three children out in Queens where the husband has AIDS and the wife is distraught. Our Buddy was once married and has two children of his own; it gives the wife a break. This sick man is so interesting. He's not admitting anything and has even told them in the hospital that he doesn't want to know what he has. But he must know. I think his wife feels he's been bisexual all along and that's where he's picked this up. Later, we find out that the family has been completely shunned by their neighbors, the children isolated on their block."

Cutler is himself "scared to death." But even before the AIDS scare began, he had begun to moderate his life. "I said to myself, 'Hey, enough of this; I'm really bored with it.' I slowed down more when I found out all this was happening. I realize that I need to be more careful. I had been very, very wild, very socially active, and just a busy bee. But I know I've had sex with men who've gotten AIDS and my own immune system isn't right. I'm terribly worried about my future. But meanwhile, I'm trying to do something that I know is important."

Cutler's group—and his feelings about what he personally is doing—are duplicated again and again across the country.

Caitlin Ryan, psychotherapist with the Whitman-Walker Clinic in Washington, describes a multitude of services to patients, their lovers, and their families, as well as to those described as "worried well," services that are being duplicated nationally, with speakers' bureaus, legal and financial services, hot lines, and educational materials now standard offerings.

But not all gay men with the disease care to participate in these activities. While the epidemic has created a new activism and sense of community, it has left many emotionally stranded; being drawn together with others as part of a disease entity is repellent and distressing to some people. A common feeling of many men was highlighted by Dr. Lawrence Mass, in an early (September 1981) article in *The New York Native*: "I think it's important for gay people not to fall into the self-hating guilt trip that we, like other minorities, have always 'fallen' into in the past."

Mea Culpa

Two Los Angeles men with Kaposi's are among many who have refused medical treatment. A combination of mistrust of the medical profession, fears of therapy further lowering their immune function, and the feeling that they have caused themselves to become ill has brought them to this decision.

"I've never come to terms with what I am," said thirty-four-year-old Bob. "My whole life has been one of control in exchange for which I've squeezed all pleasure from my life, all the humor. I've been stuck. I've built up my own business and it's successful and it doesn't mean anything to me. I've had a tremendous lot of stress the past few years and, for myself, it's been the main cause of letting my immune system break down."

Bob, a typical Southern California "health nut," has never used drugs nor been especially active sexually. He is self-contained and mature, but, he says, "I'm not taking traditional treatment because when I was diagnosed, they didn't have any answers for me and I don't intend to sap my immune system further with the kinds of treatments that are being given."

Zip is younger and sicker, the KS lesions marring his lip

and nose. "I'm full of these things, they're all down in my stomach, too," he says. He takes personal responsibility for getting AIDS and for curing himself. "I've probably never been emotionally healthy; always depressed, angry. If it hadn't been AIDS, it would have been something else, I expect."

Zip's life is different from Bob's. His parents know he is gay—he thinks—but it is an open secret about which none of them speaks. "I'm just like my mother and father; we're all secretive people. My father withdrew from us years ago and my mom turned to me as a lover—not sexually, but emotionally. I was the perfect little boy, the only son. I had to be; it's what they expected. But I've taken my father's place with my mother and it's a terrible responsibility. I'm trying to decide how I can go back and give her up, get them back together."

Zip's "secrets" are the leitmotivs of his life: "At work, I'm seen as amusing, competent, and, I think, straight. But after work—well, that's something else. I've done everything sexually. Maybe death is all that's left—the ultimate sexual experience." His profession reflects his need to "come out": Zip teaches children rendered mute by birth defects and autism how to communicate to the world.

These men, and many others, agree with New York psychologist Dr. Hal Kooden, who has written, "I view the appearance of AIDS as another example of the failure of the orthodox, medical-model approach to disease and health care." Citing the stress he and others have seen in the male homosexual community over the years, Kooden attempts various changes in overall life and health practices with his patients, and says he has seen improvement in the condition of many. "The gay man who is homophobic himself must experience some degree of bodily tension, a stress with which he lives continuously," Kooden reasons.

For many gay men, homophobic attitudes in the society

at large reflect their own negative feelings about themselves. They assign the responsibility for destructive self-images— though by no means do all gay men share them—to a hatred of homosexuals. Dr. Joel Weisman, who has been involved with AIDS since the first cases of pneumocystis were reported from his practice, emphatically agrees: "Gay coupling is very difficult in this society. It's impossible to find acceptance in middle America. And there's a hostility factor inherent in this situation. It makes for very angry sex."

Marcus Conant in San Francisco feels there are "a lot of psychological problems in the community and many men are looking for who rather than what causes AIDS. If you can blame yourself, maybe you can expunge the illness and wellness will come rushing in." Conant received a long letter written by a group of gay men and women which suggested that "gay men with AIDS are very, very serious in their dissatisfaction with typical gay sexuality which confuses impulse with compulsion."

Lesbians

As gay women are not involved in the sexual practices or diseases experienced by gay men, and only those few who use IV drugs have contracted AIDS, they are excluded from this section on homosexuality. No epidemic of sexually transmitted disease has ever been reported in the lesbian community; their rate of infection from common agents such as those that cause syphilis and gonorrhea, as well as the incidence of hepatitis and gastroenteric infection, is lower than that of heterosexual women who are sexually active. A general lack of casual sex and, as one physician put it, "not coming into contact with that great inoculum, the male penis," makes gay women among the healthiest people in the country.

Dr. Ammann says if he wanted the "cleanest possible blood" for his babies, lesbians would be the source.

Private Judgments—Public Issues

The tangle of morals and medicine that characterizes AIDS veers back and forth between those who have aligned themselves on opposite sides of the largely homophobic fence. Even those who attempt to suppress these feelings occasionally let them out in peculiar ways, as did one physician who tagged a long, neutral discussion of AIDS by quoting loosely from the Book of Leviticus: "If a man lie with another man, he shall be killed. It is an abomination in the sight of God."

Charges that the Reagan administration has dragged its feet on AIDS funding have been bolstered by Jerry Falwell, who, while designating the disease "a definite form of the judgment of God," stated that "if the Reagan administration does not put its full weight against this, what is now a gay plague in this country, I feel a year from now President Ronald Reagan personally will be blamed for allowing this awful disease to break out among the innocent American public."

Reverend William Sloane Coffin of Riverside Church in New York says flatly, "Being gay is not a sin." And the Catholic bishop of San Francisco echoes this, but adds that the sexual *acts* of homosexuals are sinful if performed.

"Can you imagine anything this straight, white, conservative cold administration would rather see than all gay men being wiped from the face of the earth?" asks a gay New York physician. This kind of feeling of being under siege leads to uncomfortable speculation about elaborate "genocide" plots and notions like "ethnic-chemical weapons"—described in the book *A Higher Form of Killing*: "[Those] would be designed to exploit naturally occurring differences in vulnerability among specific population groups."

But AIDS cannot be said to have been the sole reason that gay sexuality has become a political issue. When physicians are reluctant to advise their patients on ways to prevent or reduce illness—as has been the case for those treating gay men whose sexual activities keep them constantly infected—there is an a priori political implication.

Dr. Bob Bolan of San Francisco says, "I would have been stoned to death by my colleagues a year ago for suggesting that the behaviors that led to illness bordered on addictive-type behavior."

New York dermatologist Patrick Hennessey now advises patients to "basically not have anonymous sex—or much of any kind of sex except monogamous. Even a year ago I would have been uncomfortable saying that."

Dan William says that physicians have in the past helped reinforce the misconception that "personal choice left solely to the judgment of the individual (which often entailed multiple infections) was an acceptable health risk." But Joel Weisman emphatically states that "it took this kind of crisis to be able to tell people—'Cool it!' "

Why would physicians seeing the health consequences of multiple sex encounters be unable to speak of their concerns to their patients? It appears that the liberated gay life-style has been seen as a brave standard carried by a few and that to suggest another mode of behavior—regardless of the reasons for so doing—would have appeared to be a " 'judgmental' affront to the 'gay rights' movement," as Jonathan Lieberson put it in *The New York Review of Books*. Even those doctors and gay men who have perceived the practices of the "bathhouse culture" as dangerous or aberrant have been firm in their insistence that it is the right of gay men to conduct themselves as they see fit.

D. H. Lawrence said that "sin isn't the breaking of Divine

Commandments. It is the breaking of one's own integrity."
Each societal group establishes the parameters of its own "integrity"; it appears that many of the problems and conflicts
in the gay community stem from the fact that no clear consensus has been reached on the parameters of its integrity.

Roger Enlow reports that early in the AIDS epidemic,
some thought was given to a voluntary withdrawal of blood
donations by gay men until the mode of transmission was
firmly established. But the idea was put aside, as many felt
it would imply an acceptance that *their* blood was "bad" and
was causing AIDS.

No agreement has been reached on an acceptable degree
of candor regarding gay sex practices. What effect would such
facts have on the public? Would it tend to take some of the
mystery away from gay life? Or would it reinforce homophobia? Many homosexuals feel that the attitude held by most
gay men—that sex has nothing to do with morals—would
largely be incomprehensible and unacceptable to the majority
of Americans.

One of Lawrence Mass's patients is quoted as saying that
there is a "Catch-22" in society's perception of gays. "It says
because homosexuals are promiscuous, immature, and incapable of forming stable relationships, they are therefore forbidden the legal, theological, and social opportunities to
establish them." On the other hand, he continues, many straight
people "who decry promiscuity are equally contemptuous of
gay love relationships that are monogamous. They don't draw
distinctions."

Conclusion

When the idea of writing this book first came up in the fall of 1981, the inclination was to follow the investigation of the disease and, when the cause and cure were found, to have at hand a summation of its history with which to formulate a medical mystery story with a beginning, middle, and end. But although a probable agent has been found, the story has no denouement, no ending; the elements do not fall into neat, easy patterns.

Instead of a complete story, then, we have compiled an account that includes much guesswork and speculation. We have been obliged to end too many sentences and chapters with question marks instead of statements of fact. As bizarre as it seems in this day of scientific miracles, it may take years or "forever" to find a vaccine or treatment for AIDS.

Scientists are now entering pre-AIDS patients in five-year studies; research tracks are being diverted to work on AIDS (not a simple matter of moving test tubes from one bench to another). Worst-case scenarios project 3.3 million cases of AIDS and 1.6 million fatalities by 1988. In the summer of 1983, Marc Conant told a congressional committee: "If I put a vaccine in front of you today and we began, it would make no impact on the disease until at least 1985. Every case that is going to appear by then is already in the pipeline and we have no way of stopping it."

Jim Curran of the CDC counters what he sees as dooms-day predictions by saying: "Mathematical projections that AIDS will soon hit vastly larger numbers of people are irresponsible. It's reasonable to suggest that cases will continue to increase this year, but why not project up to the year 2100 and say everyone in the world will have it?" Of course, Jim Curran is right. An organism, unless programmed for total destruc-tion—including self-destruction—does not completely de-stroy its own environment. Who could imagine that a single strand of RNA would formulate a biologic final solution?

Instead, though at the cost of thousands of innocent lives—and, regardless of what one may feel about gays or junkies or Haitian illegal immigrants, they are all as innocent as pedes-trians run down on the sidewalk by a berserk tanker truck—AIDS is presenting scientists with a living experiment of na-ture in which what we don't know will become known. As cold-blooded as that seems, it is a perfectly acceptable, rea-sonable way—the only way we have—to study the human in health and disease.

"The study of AIDS absolutely is going to give us im-portant information about how the immune system is regu-lated," says Dr. Cunningham-Rundles. "This will be valuable ultimately not only to AIDS patients: it will help us to design therapy for cancer patients who have a secondary immune deficiency as a result of radiation therapy or chemotherapy or a large tumor burden."

But the potential payoff from AIDS research is far greater. Maybe solving the AIDS puzzle will mean we won't have any more cancer patients to treat. The "immune surveillance" theory that has been as much poetic fantasy as it has been scientific fact may now begin to be illuminated enough so that we will be able to prevent, instead of treat, cancers. AIDS seems to validate the theory; AIDS is showing us what may well be cancer in an epidemic, viral form.

Research into AIDS will elucidate the mechanisms of autoimmune diseases, perhaps establish a viral genesis for multiple sclerosis, rheumatoid arthritis, and a hundred other presently incurable illnesses. The dysfunction that follows with AIDS goes to the heart of life and watches DNA and perhaps RNA viral entities play trade-off with our individual genetic material.

AIDS suggests that certain groups of people have inherited or developed immune configurations that, though adequate in normal circumstances, leave gay men, Haitians, perhaps hemophiliacs open for its particular effects.

It is reasonable to assume that even if we are not able to prevent or cure AIDS, we will soon be able to at least keep alive those afflicted by the disease. But this begs a question perhaps larger than the illness itself: Does the United States want to invest vast sums of money for the protection of those in the groups that are the prime targets of the disease? Will homophobia, and the generalized fear of "others" in this country, allow for such drains on an already overburdened health system to care for outcasts? Or do we let them die?

AIDS may have already made these questions academic. Roger Enlow thinks the disease marks a watershed in the affairs of homosexual people in America. For the first time their leaders are recognized, are able to make appointments with Cabinet-level leaders; homosexuals are acknowledged to be a specific constituency. If, as is estimated, 25 million U.S.

citizens are homosexual—and if they have a perception of how the country should approach their needs—the realities of AIDS may turn their inchoate desires into a political consensus. They may start to have a serious impact on the social process.

Certainly, gay men are being forced by AIDS to reorganize their personal priorities, to put aside self-preoccupation and to turn their abilities outward to the good of a wider community. And many express relief that they have been "let off the hook" of sexual excesses that go against their personal beliefs and private sense of self. If sexuality has been a statement of gay freedom, and that statement has turned out to be a death sentence, how will gays redirect their energies?

Forty percent of all AIDS victims in the United States are black or Hispanic. Though this fact has largely been ignored thus far, it underlies the overall epidemic and sooner or later will have to be addressed by those groups.

AIDS has also revealed weaknesses in our health-care and research funding mechanisms. The slowness of the Department of Health and Human Services in responding to the emergency, the National Institutes of Health's inability to meet emergencies, the overburdening of an underfunded Centers for Disease Control—all these institutional problems will now come under scrutiny. Most telling, we have discovered anew the lack of readiness by the federal government to aid citizens laid low by an emergency disease situation. If AIDS does nothing but stimulate a search for solutions to this inadequacy, major good will have come from this evil.

The epidemic also has thrown light on this country's enormous traffic in the buying and selling of human blood. America buys and sells half of all blood that is used medically. Serious questions have arisen as to the quality of oversight, control, and safety procedures with regard to the "blood industry."

AIDS fear, combined with endemic venereal herpes, the upsurge of drug-resistant gonorrhea, the prevalence of hepatitis B—all sexually transmitted—surely will moderate the sexual "swinging" of the 1970s and early 1980s among Americans of all sexual preferences. Who could not become more modest in the face of such a magnitude of disease?

Unfortunately, there is one group that likely will ignore these realities and that may well constitute the final and most numerous victims as time passes. Unreachable through reason or census, IV drug users are already so far outside the mainstream, so addicted to a lawless existence that their numbers may be the AIDS reservoir of tomorrow.

AIDS started as an "American" disease. But it is spreading in Europe and across central Africa. What will be the reaction of our friends to our part in the promulgation of this deadly syndrome among them? Dr. M. A. Epstein, co-discoverer of the Epstein-Barr virus, remarked at a press conference in New York, "Perhaps AIDS is Africa taking revenge for the slave trade." An unfortunate "joke," he later explained.

"I used to be totally confident," scientist and writer Dr. Lewis Thomas has said, "that the great infectious diseases of humankind were completely under control and would soon, maybe in my own lifetime, vanish as threats to human health." But the advent of AIDS has forced Dr. Thomas to disavow that confident belief. "We are not about to finish the job in infectious disease, nor are we likely to in the near term, maybe not in the long term."

The great advances of modern medical science may have led many of us, along with Dr. Thomas, into false complacency. Polio and measles and smallpox can be prevented; pneumonia and tuberculosis successfully treated. We can transplant organs, reattach severed limbs, and restore the sight of many who are blind. But with the appearance of a new epidemic such as AIDS, we are reminded that there have been many diseases of epidemic proportion through history that appeared suddenly, ravaged a population, and eventually disappeared—leaving scientists baffled. Thucydides faithfully recorded every symptom of an epidemic that killed thousands of Greeks and their enemies, yet no scientist has ever identified the disease, nor has its equivalent ever reappeared. Following the worldwide epidemic of influenza after World War I (an epidemic that is thought to have taken between 20 and 30 million lives), another illness (probably related to that flu) made its appearance—an infection of the brain that caused Parkinson's disease; the causative agent has never been identified.

It could well turn out that, despite the great advances in medical knowledge, expertise, and technologies, AIDS will join the ranks of the great mystery diseases of history.

Though the shortsighted will continue to think of this disease as something that "kills queers," AIDS is an important event in this country's history as well as in world science. How we manage it will say much about our validity as humans in the history books of the future.

Glossary

Acquired Immune Deficiency Syndrome (AIDS): A disease characterized by failure of the immune system to protect against infections and certain cancers. This defect strikes previously healthy individuals who have no known cause for the immunosuppression. It is not inherited (hence the word "acquired"). First described in mid-1981. Cause(s), prevention, and cure unknown.

African Connection: Refers to the speculation that AIDS possibly arose in Africa.

Allergens: Substances that cause allergic reactions; e.g., grass and tree pollen.

Allergy: An immunologically mediated sensitivity to foreign substances, which may cause various symptoms; e.g., sneezing, rash, and difficulty breathing.

Amyl nitrite: An inhalable fluorocarbon that dilates the blood vessels.

Antibiotics: Drugs that help the body resist infection by bacteria, fungi, protozoa, or other microorganisms.

Antibody: A protein that specifically combines with and helps to destroy a foreign substance in the body. Antibodies are manufactured by B-lymphocytes in response to the presence of specific antigens. Once an antibody is formed, the cell has a "memory" of the event; this "memory" renders the patient immune to that specific antigen in the future.

256

Antigen: A substance that is recognized as foreign by the immune system. Specific substances, called antigen receptors, are found on the surfaces of both B-lymphocytes and T-lymphocytes. These antigen receptors make possible the reaction of B- and T-lymphocytes to antigens. Without antigen receptors, the lymphocytes cannot respond to the presence of antigens and no immune response takes place.

Antigenic overload: See *immune overload.*

Antihistamine: A drug that helps to block the effects of the natural substance histamine, which mediates allergic reactions.

Apheresis: A technique in which the blood is circulated outside the body and certain components are removed. In plasmapheresis the liquid portion of the blood is removed and the cells returned. In lymphapheresis the lymphocytes are removed and the liquid portion of the blood returned to the subject's body. In leukapheresis all white blood cells are removed. In some diseases plasmapheresis is thought to remove toxic substances that promote disease.

Arthritis: Inflammation of the joints and/or muscles. A symptom of more than one hundred diseases.

Autoimmune disease: A condition in which a person's immune system perceives the body's own cells as foreign and attacks them.

B-lymphocyte: A lymphocyte that produces antibodies to create immunity against certain diseases. Antibodies are important for protection against bacterial infection, for example.

Bacteremia: The presence in the blood of living bacteria.

Bacterium: A small, simple, single-celled organism. Many forms of bacteria are capable of causing illness.

Biopsy: A surgical procedure to remove a small sample of tissue in order to examine it in the laboratory to assist in making a diagnosis.

Bisexual: A sexual orientation in which a person enjoys having sex with both men and women.

Bone marrow: The substance that produces blood cells. Found in the hollow center of the long bones of the arms and legs.

Brain tumor: An abnormal growth in the brain; can be benign or cancerous.

Burkitt's lymphoma: A cancer of the lymphatic tissue thought to be associated with Epstein-Barr virus. Mainly affects children in equatorial Africa.

Cachexia: A state of profound metabolic disorder and wasting. Can be a result of malnutrition. Often associated with cancer.

Cancer: Abnormal growth of tissues that can spread to different parts of the body. These distant colonies are called metastases.

Candidiasis: Infection with a yeastlike fungus called candida. When this organism is present in the throat and mouth the condition is called thrush.

Case-control study: An epidemiologic method in which persons with a disease condition are compared to a healthy population similar in age, sex, race, etc., to determine how the ill persons differ from a healthy population. Often useful in identifying factors that may contribute to a disease state.

CDC criteria: The specific criteria by which CDC defines an individual case of illness as AIDS. The CDC definition requires that a person have an illness strongly suggestive of an underlying immune deficit, such as opportunistic infections or Kaposi's sarcoma, in the absence of any treatment or disease condition that suppresses the immune system.

Cell: The smallest independent unit of an organism. A cell is composed of cytoplasm and a nucleus and is surrounded by a membrane.

Cell-mediated immunity: Immunity conferred by the T-lymphocytes.

Chemotherapy: Treatment of a disease with chemicals, such as antibiotics or cytotoxic drugs.

Chromosome: Structures containing genetic material (DNA) within the nucleus of cells.

Cimetidine: A drug that is used to treat ulcers. It also has effects on the immune system and is being investigated as one adjunct therapy for AIDS.

Circulating immune complexes: Immune complexes found in blood when antigens are present in excess amounts. Can cause diseases, such as nephritis and kidney failure.

Clone: A group of cells derived from a single parent cell and identical to it.

Clotting factors: Substances in the blood essential for the normal coagulation of blood.

CMV: See *cytomegalovirus.*

Congenital: Any condition present at birth. Opposite of "acquired."

Constitutional symptoms: In AIDS, any one of a group of clinical symptoms thought to be indicative of an early stage of AIDS. These include malaise, fatigue, diarrhea, fever, night sweats, and severe weight loss over a period of months.

Corticosteroids: Natural substances that function as hormones in the body and are used as pharmacologic agents to treat many inflammatory diseases, such as arthritis.

Cryptococcus: A fungus that rarely causes infection in healthy persons. One of the opportunistic infections found in AIDS patients.

Cytomegalovirus (CMV): A herpes virus commonly found in AIDS patients and also in otherwise healthy homosexuals. CMV is capable of producing serious illness in infants, weakened persons, and those whose immune systems have been suppressed by drugs or cancer.

Cytotoxic drugs: Chemical substances having a toxic or killing effect on cells.

DNA: The double helix of genetic material that carries the genetic information.

Encephalitis: Inflammation of the brain; usually caused by a viral infection.

Endemic: A condition or disease that is widespread in a population. Compare *epidemic.*

Endoscopy: The passage of a tube into the stomach or intestine through which the interior of those organs can be viewed to aid medical diagnosis or treatment.

Enteritis: Inflammation of the intestines, particularly the small intestine.

Epidemic: An outbreak of a disease among a population that is not normally found in a large fraction of that population. Compare *endemic.*

Epidemiology: The discipline of tracking and discovering the cause(s) of an epidemic.

Epstein-Barr virus (EBV): A virus responsible for infectious mononucleosis and implicated in Burkitt's lymphoma. Found in a high percentage of gay men. EBV is in the herpes virus family.

Factor VIII: One of the clotting factors in the blood. Congenital absence of Factor VIII causes a disease called hemophilia A.

Gamma globulin: A family of serum proteins containing the antibodies.

Gastroenteritis: Inflammation of the lining of the stomach and intestine.

Gay bowel syndrome: A disease condition in which a person has repeated bouts of diarrhea due to infection with parasites such as giardia. This is called "gay" bowel syndrome because the sexual practices of gay men make them especially prone to this disease.

Genetic marker: Any substance that can be measured and whose presence is an indicator of an inherited disorder.

Giardia: An intestinal parasite that can cause severe diarrhea and stomach pain. One of the organisms in the gay bowel syndrome.

Gland: An organ that produces a specialized substance necessary for physiology, such as a hormone, that is released into the blood to act at a distant site.

Hemolytic anemia: A disease in which the red blood cells are destroyed at an increased rate.

Hemophilia: A genetic disorder of males characterized by an inability of the blood to clot properly. The cause is an absence of a clotting factor called Factor VIII.

Hepatitis: An inflammation of the liver. It can be caused by one of several viruses: hepatitis A (primarily spread through feces), hepatitis B (primarily spread through blood transfusion), and non-A, non-B hepatitis (also spread through blood transfusion). Hepatitis A mostly causes acute illness, often subclinical in the young and more severe in the elderly. Hepatitis B can cause either acute or chronic illness and is associated with liver cancer. It induces a carrier state in about 10 percent of patients: they are not ill, but can transmit the disease (by blood transfusions, from mother to newborn, or through saliva, breast milk, or genital secretions).

Herpes simplex: A herpes virus that causes mostly self-healing cold sores, usually around the mouth and genital area. Often transmitted by sexual contact. In AIDS severe untreatable herpes simplex blisters have occurred in the anal area in some patients.

Herpes virus: A family of viruses that are large, are covered by a fatty envelope, and contain a large amount of DNA as their genetic material. They include herpes simplex, herpes zoster, Epstein-Barr virus, and cytomegalovirus. Herpes viruses tend to occur in a severe form in immunocompromised patients, such as those with AIDS.

Herpes zoster: The herpes virus that causes chicken pox. It also causes shingles, a painful blistering inflammation around the trunk of the body. In immunosuppressed patients, such as those with AIDS and cancer patients, the herpes zoster virus can cause infection throughout the body.

Histocompatibility antigens (HLA): A group of substances (human leukocyte antigens) found on the membranes of cells that are characteristic of the genetic history of a person. They are identified to determine the compatibility of tissues or organs such as kidneys for transplant procedures. There is some evidence of an HLA-linked genetic factor in AIDS patients that is not present in non-AIDS individuals.

Histoplasmosis: A fungal disease of the lungs.

Hodgkin's lymphoma: One kind of cancer of the lymphatic system.

Host defense: The sum of all bodily protections against disease. Host defense starts with the physical barrier to infection provided by the skin and continues to cells called macrophages, which engulf invaders, and other types of nonspecific protection. The immune system is an integral part of host defense.

HTLV (human T-cell leukemia virus): A recently identified virus associated with certain types of leukemia endemic in specific geographic areas such as southern Japan and the Caribbean. A possible association of HTLV with AIDS is currently being explored.

HTLV-III (Human T-cell lymphatrophic virus): Thought to be a member of the same retroviral family, this virus, discovered in 1983, is believed by many to be the cause or a cofactor in AIDS.

Humoral immunity: The resistance to disease conferred by the antibodies produced by the B-lymphocytes.

Immune complex: A large molecule containing a number of antibodies and antigens combined. See *circulating immune complexes.*

Immune overload: In AIDS, the theory that the breakdown of the immune system is caused by years of multiple recurrent infections that somehow cause the immune system to cease functioning properly.

Immune system: A complex of cells and proteins that helps fight infectious diseases and possibly also cancer.

Immunization: Protection against disease by vaccination or inoculation, usually by introduction of a weakened form of the infectious agent or of a component of the organism that cannot cause disease by itself.

Immunocompromised: The state of improper function of the immune system. See *immunodeficiency.*

Immunodeficiency: A state in which the immune system does not function properly. It is marked by repeated severe infections and, in extreme cases, by an increased incidence of certain cancers. Immunodeficiency can be inherited, in which case it is called congenital immunodeficiency, or caused after birth, called acquired immunodeficiency. Acquired immunodeficiency can be brought on by disease, such as cancer, or by medical treatment, such as drugs used to prevent transplant rejection. An acquired immunodeficiency of unknown cause underlies the many manifestations of AIDS.

Immunoglobulins: The serum proteins that confer immunity. The three most common types are immunoglobulin G (IgG), immunoglobulin M (IgM), and immunoglobulin A (IgA).

Immunology: The study of the immune system and its diseases.

Immunosuppressive drugs: Chemicals that lower immune activity. Some are designed to treat various illnesses in which the immune system is overactive, such as lupus. Others are used to prevent rejection of transplanted organs. Still others are used to destroy tumors and suppress immunity as an unwanted side effect.

Incubation time: The period between exposure to an infectious agent and the first signs of the infection.

Infectious mononucleosis: An acute viral infection with Epstein-Barr virus. Also known as the "kissing disease," because it can be transmitted by intimate contact, and "glandular fever," because it involves swelling of the lymph nodes.

Interferons: Chemical substances produced by cells in response to infection. There are now known to be at least fifty different types of interferons. These natural hormones are thought to be involved in the regulation of the immune system. Interferons are being tested for cancer chemotherapy, as well as for their ability to restore the immune system in patients with AIDS.

Interleukin-2 (IL2): A chemical substance thought to regulate the production and maturation of many types of T-lymphocytes and B-lymphocytes.

Isolate: A strain of a microorganism grown from the tissues of a person with an infectious disease.

Isolation: A medical precaution in which patients with a contagious infectious disease are kept separate from healthy persons or from other patients who do not have that particular disease.

Kaposi's sarcoma (KS): A cancer of the blood vessels that usually appears first on the skin. It is common in equatorial Africa, where it often has an aggressive course and even affects children. In the United States it is mostly found among elderly men of Mediterranean descent, in whom it progresses slowly, rarely kills, and can be treated. As one of the manifestations of AIDS, Kaposi's sarcoma strikes young men and is intermediate in virulence between the African and classical American diseases. Cytomegalovirus may be involved in this cancer.

Killer T-lymphocytes: These are lymphocytes that come into contact with foreign cells, tumor cells, and cells infected with viruses, and kill them.

Latency: The period between contracting a disease and showing the first symptoms. Similar to the incubation period. In AIDS, the latency period is quite long, apparently between six months and perhaps more than two years.

LAV: Lymphadenopathy-associated virus.

Legionnaire's disease: An acute infectious pneumonia caused by a water-borne bacterium.

Lesion: Any abnormality of a tissue or organ. A lesion can be a visible change or a metabolic abnormality.

Leukemia: A cancer of the white blood cells and bone marrow.

Leukocytes: White blood cells. Three types of leukocytes are macrophages, lymphocytes, and polymorphonuclear leukocytes.

Leukopenia: A condition in which there are too few white blood cells.

Lyme arthritis: A recently identified inflammatory disease caused by a bacterium transmitted by the bite of a tick.

Lymph nodes: Small collections of tissue that contain large numbers of lymphocytes and capture foreign particles and cells carried in the lymph. In AIDS, the architecture and cellular composition of the lymph nodes is altered.

Lymphadenopathy: Persistent swelling of the lymph nodes. In AIDS, a condition of long-term generalized lymph-node swelling thought to be in some instances an early sign of infection with the putative AIDS agent. Also called lymphadenopathy syndrome (LAS).

Lymphapheresis: See *apheresis.*

Lymphocyte: A small type of white blood cell responsible for immunity. Lymphocytes originate in the bone marrow, pass through the bloodstream, and enter other organs (such as the thymus) where they become modified to T-lymphocytes and B-lymphocytes.

Lymphokines: Substances released by T-lymphocytes that assist in the immune response. Two lymphokines are interferon and interleukin-2.

Lymphoma: Cancer of the lymphoid tissues.

Lymphopenia: An abnormally low number of lymphocytes.

Macrophage: From the Greek words for "big" and "eater." A white blood cell that destroys foreign substances and cells. It also cooperates with T- and B-lymphocytes in the immune response.

Memory cells: T-lymphocytes that have been exposed to specific antigens and are capable of proliferating and mounting a rapid immune response upon a repeat encounter with those antigens.

Meningitis: Inflammation of the membranes that cover the brain and spinal cord. Most commonly caused by viral and bacterial infections.

Metabolism: The chemical processes that take place in the body.

Microbes: Microscopic organisms.

Minor AIDS: Also called "lesser AIDS." The term used by some to refer to symptoms that may signal the early phase of infection with the putative AIDS agent. In most cases minor AIDS does not appear to go on to "full-blown AIDS." See *constitutional symptoms*. Compare *prodrome*.

Mitogen response: A proliferative response of T-lymphocytes to a nonspecific stimulus in the test tube. In immunodeficient patients the mitogen response is decreased.

Monoclonal: Derived from one group of cells or organisms, all having the same ancestry and therefore all identical.

Monoclonal antibody: A homogeneous antibody produced by the fusion of a B-lymphocyte and a cancer cell. Used to identify specific blood cells, such as T-helper lymphocytes and T-suppressor lymphocytes.

Mutation: A change in genetic information, either spontaneous or caused by an external event.

Mycobacterium: A bacterium possessing a waxy outer capsule. These organisms cause pneumonia.

Myeloma: A cancer growth of antibody-producing cells in the bone marrow.

Neoplastic: A term that refers to tissues that are proliferating inappropriately or in an uncontrolled fashion. The tissue is called a neoplasm or a tumor. When a neoplasm invades nearby tissues or spreads to other parts of the body it is called malignant or cancerous.

Nonsteroidal antiinflammatory drugs (NSAIDS): Drugs that reduce inflammation. See *prostaglandins*.

Nucleus: The part of the cell that contains the DNA.

Oncogenic: Able to cause tumors.

Opportunistic infection (OI): Any infection that is caused by a microorganism commonly found in the environment but that causes disease only in persons who are weakened or whose immune systems are deficient. These infections are frequently the immediate cause of death in AIDS patients, though the underlying "cause" is the immune deficiency.

Papovavirus: A family of small viruses that contains DNA as the hereditary material and includes the viruses that cause warts. A member of this family also causes a brain disease called progressive multifocal leukoencephalopathy, which has been found in some AIDS patients.

Parasite: Microorganism that conducts its life cycle inside a host's cells.

Parvovirus: A family of small DNA-containing viruses known to cause illness in cats, dogs, and cows.

Passive immunity: Transfer of immune leukocytes or gamma globulin containing antibodies from one person to another.

Pentamidine: An antibiotic used in the treatment of pneumonia caused by pneumocystis carinii.

Plasma: The fluid part of the blood. Contains the proteins and minerals.

Plasma cell: The mature B-lymphocyte that produces antibodies.

Plasmapheresis: See *apheresis.*

Platelets: The blood particles that play an important part in the clotting of blood.

Pneumocystis carinii pneumonia (PCP): A form of pneumonia caused by a protozoan parasite. It usually does not cause an infection in a host with an intact immune system. This organism is the most common one isolated in AIDS patients and is associated with a high death rate in AIDS.

Polyclonal: Having an origin in more than one ancestor. Compare *monoclonal.*

Prodrome: A group of symptoms that appears in an individual before the full manifestation of an illness. In AIDS, physicians so far prefer the term "lesser AIDS" for the constitutional symptoms that are thought to signal the early stages of AIDS, because most of these patients do not go on to develop "full-blown AIDS."

Prostaglandins: A group of chemicals made by platelets and other cells in the body that affect many different functions. Prostaglandins are involved in causing inflammation, and aspirin and nonsteroidal antiinflammatory drugs act by inhibiting production of prostaglandins.

Proteins: Organic compounds composed of amino acids that are necessary for life. Some proteins, called enzymes, carry out metabolism, while others make up antibodies, and still others act as structural elements of cells.

Protozoan: One type of parasite.

Radiation therapy: Treatment of cancer with a beam or other intense source of radiation.

Radioimmunoassay: A very sensitive test employing radioactive compounds and antibodies that measures the presence of a variety of substances in the blood.

Retrovirus: A virus containing RNA as the genetic material that causes cancers in animals. HTLV is the first retrovirus shown to cause cancer in humans.

Risk factor: Any personal or environmental condition that increases an individual's probability of getting a disease.

RNA: A form of genetic material complementary to DNA.

Sedimentation rate: The rate at which red blood cells go to the bottom of a test tube under increased centrifugal force. An altered sedimentation rate is a general sign of illness and accompanies many diseases.

Serum: The clear fluid that remains after the cells are removed from blood and the resulting plasma is allowed to clot.

Severe combined immunodeficiency syndrome: A severe inherited immune deficiency disease in which both humoral and cell-mediated immunity are absent.

Spectrum: In infectious diseases, the range of severity of disease, ranging from infection without symptoms to lethal illness. Many researchers think this concept accurately describes the range of conditions seen among those at risk for AIDS. See *prodrome, minor AIDS, lymphadenopathy, constitutional symptoms.*

Steroids: See *corticosteroids.*

Surveillance: In immunology, the process by which the immune system monitors the presence of foreign organisms or abnormal cells, such as tumor cells, in the body. In epidemiology, the process of identifying all the cases of a given illness for study.

T-helper lymphocytes: Those T-lymphocytes that assist B-lymphocytes in maturing to produce antibody and that enhance cell-mediated immunity.

T-lymphocyte: One type of lymphocyte; responsible for protecting against a range of infectious agents, particularly those that replicate inside cells, such as viruses, parasites, and fungi. T-lymphocytes also regulate the functions of a variety of other cells of the immune system. See also *B-lymphocyte, killer T-lymphocytes, lymphocyte, T-suppressor lymphocytes.*

T-suppressor lymphocytes: A subgroup of T-lymphocytes that regulate immune functions, such as antibody production by B-lymphocytes. Some T-suppressor lymphocytes may express cytotoxic T-lymphocyte activity.

Thrombocytopenia: A deficiency of thrombocytes, also called platelets, the small cell fragments that are essential to clotting of blood. One of the occasional manifestations of AIDS is a condition called idiopathic thrombocytopenic purpura (ITP), a decrease in platelet number probably due to antibody produced against them. It leads to uncontrolled bleeding. It is another manifestation of the disorder in regulation of B-lymphocytes that is part of AIDS.

Thrush: A fungal infection of the mouth and throat caused by the fungus candida.

Thymosin: A hormone produced by the thymus gland that regulates the immune system. Used in the treatment of immune deficiency diseases, including AIDS.

Thymus gland: A small gland in the chest that regulates the development of T-lymphocytes and makes hormones that are important in maintaining proper immunity.

Toxoplasmosis: Infectious disease caused by the protozoan parasite toxoplasma gondii. Seldom causes disease in healthy people, but toxoplasmosis of the brain has commonly been found as a concomitant of AIDS among Haitians.

Transfusion: Using whole blood to replace or augment blood or blood components in persons undergoing surgery, those with blood loss, or patients with specific deficits in the blood.

Tumor: Any abnormal growth, whether a danger to health or not. Compare *cancer, neoplastic.*

Ulcer: An eroded portion on the skin or mucous membrane that exposes underlying tissues.

Vaccine: A suspension of weakened or killed virus or bacteria that is administered to protect against illness caused by those microorganisms. See *immunization.*

Virus: A subcellular microorganism composed of genetic material, either DNA or RNA, and protein. In the body, viruses multiply only within host cells.

Annotated Selected Bibliography

Reports and information about AIDS come from many sources, including science magazines, general-interest magazines, and medical journals. The following lists provide an overview of the available sources.

Extensive Bibliographies

The National Institute of Allergy and Infectious Diseases AIDS Bibliography. This bibliography includes articles in medical journals, magazines, and major newspapers. It is indexed by topic and updated frequently. Free copies are sent to "individual scientists and clinicians and interested organizations." Write to:

> AIDS Bibliography
> NIAID
> 9000 Rockville Pike
> Building 5, Room 135
> Bethesda, MD 20205

Gays and Acquired Immune Deficiency Syndrome: A Bibliography, compiled by Alan V. Miller (Toronto: Canadian Gay Archives). This is periodically updated, so ask for the latest edition.

Important Journal Articles

Major research reports of AIDS appear frequently in the following journals:

>*Annals of Internal Medicine*
>*Cancer*
>*Cancer Research*
>*Cancer Treatment Reports*
>*The Journal of the American Medical Association*
>*Lancet*
>*Nature*
>*New England Journal of Medicine*
>*Science*

Morbidity and Mortality Reports

This weekly newsletter published by the Centers for Disease Control carried the initial reports of the illness that would become known as AIDS as well as notification of each new risk group and significant findings about the syndrome. The brief, almost telegraphic articles make up the progress notes of the AIDS investigation.

Gay Press

Some of the most interesting articles pertaining to the social and emotional facets of AIDS have appeared in the gay press. Many are written by physicians on the medical aspects as well. The following have published hundreds of articles on the disease:

>*Advocate* (Los Angeles)
>*Bay Area Reporter* (San Francisco)
>*The Body Politic* (Toronto)
>*Christopher Street* (New York)
>*Gay Community News* (Boston)
>*Gay News* (Philadelphia)
>*GayLife* (Chicago)
>*In Touch* (Los Angeles)
>*New York Native* (New York)
>*Out* (Pittsburgh)
>*Washington Blade* (Washington, D.C.)

Sources

The following doctors, researchers, and lay people participated in personal interviews and/or are quoted in this book.

David Aaronson, M.D.—Chief, Coagulation Section, National Center for Drugs and Biologics, Food and Drug Administration, Bethesda, Maryland

Donald Abrams, M.D.—Assistant Physician, San Francisco General Hospital, San Francisco

Louis Aledort, M.D.—Professor of Medicine, Mt. Sinai School of Medicine, New York

Arthur J. Ammann, M.D.—Director of Research, Genetech, San Francisco

Donald Armstrong, M.D.—Chief of Infectious Diseases, Memorial Sloan-Kettering Cancer Center, New York

David Auerbach, M.D.—Fellow, Department of Medicine, University of California, Los Angeles

David Baltimore, M.D.—Director, Whitehead Institute for Biomedical Research, New York

Robert Biggar, M.D.—Medical Epidemiologist, Environmental Epidemiology, National Cancer Institute, Bethesda, Maryland

William Blattner, M.D.—Chief, Family Studies, National Cancer Institute, Bethesda, Maryland

William Boggs—Public Health Director, Krome Avenue Detention Center, Miami

Robert Bolan, M.D.—Medical Director, Gay Clinic, Presbyterian Medical Center, San Francisco

Ary Bordes, M.D.—Former Minister of Health, Haiti

Joseph Bove, M.D.—Director, Blood Banks, Yale University Hospitals, New Haven, Connecticut

Edward Brandt, M.D.—Assistant Secretary, Department of Health and Human Services, Washington, D.C.

Nathan Clumeck, M.D.—St. Pierre Hospital, Brussels, Belgium

Nancy Cole—Board of Directors, AIDS Project, Los Angeles

Jean-Claude Compas, M.D.—Chairman, Haitian Medical Association Abroad, New York

Marcus Conant, M.D.—Codirector, Kaposi's Clinic, University of California, San Francisco

Susanna Cunningham-Rundles, Ph.D.—Research Associate, Memorial Sloan-Kettering Cancer Center, New York

James E. Curran, M.D.—Coordinator, AIDS Activity, Centers for Disease Control, Atlanta

Mitchell Cutler—Coordinator, Support Services, Gay Men's Health Crisis, New York

William Darrow, Ph.D.—Research Sociologist, AIDS Activity, Centers for Disease Control, Atlanta

Jan Desmyter, M.D.—Katholieri Universiteit Te Leuven, Rega Instituut, Belgium

W. Lawrence Drew, M.D.—Director of Microbiology and Infectious Diseases, Mt. Zion Hospital, San Francisco

Selma Dritz, M.D., M.Ph.—Assistant Director, Bureau of Communicable Disease Control, Department of Public Health, San Francisco

Peter Drotman, M.D.—AIDS Activity, Centers for Disease Control, Atlanta

Roger Enlow, M.D.—Former Director, Office of Gay and Lesbian Health Concerns, Department of Public Health, City of New York

M. A. Epstein, M.D.—University of Bristol, England

Bruce Evatt, M.D.—Director, Division of Host Factors, Centers for Disease Control, Atlanta

Anthony S. Fauci, M.D.—Chief, Laboratory of Immunoregulation, National Institute of Allergy and Infectious Diseases, Bethesda, Maryland

Margaret Fischl, M.D.—Assistant Professor of Medicine, University of Miami; Director, Miami AIDS Task Force, Miami

William Foege, M.D.—Former Director, Centers for Disease Control, Atlanta

Daniel Fountain, M.D., MPH—Chef du Zone, Bandundu, Vanga, Zaire

Donald Francis, M.D.—Coordinator, AIDS Laboratory Activity, Centers for Disease Control, Atlanta

Gerald H. Friedland, M.D.—Associate Professor of Medicine, Albert Einstein College of Medicine, New York

Alvin E. Friedman-Kien, M.D.—Professor of Dermatology and Microbiology, New York University School of Medicine, New York

Robert C. Gallo, M.D.—Chief, Laboratory of Tumor Cell Biology, National Cancer Institute, Bethesda, Maryland

Edward P. Gelmann, M.D.—Laboratory of Tumor Cell Biology, National Cancer Institute, Bethesda, Maryland

Norman Geschwind, M.D.—Chairman, Department of Neurology, Harvard University Medical School, Cambridge

James Goedert, M.D.—Environmental Epidemiology, National Cancer Institute, Bethesda, Maryland

Jonathan W. Gold, M.D.—Associate Director, Special Microbiology Laboratory, Memorial Sloan-Kettering Cancer Center, New York

Allan L. Goldstein, Ph.D.—Chairman, Department of Biochemistry, George Washington University School of Medicine, Washington, D.C.

A. Arthur Gottlieb, M.D.—Tulane Medical School, New Orleans, Louisiana

Michael S. Gottlieb, M.D.—Assistant Professor of Medicine, Division of Clinical Immunology and Allergy, University of California School of Medicine, Los Angeles

Michael H. Grieco, M.D.—Director, R. A. Cooke Institute of Allergy, St. Luke's–Roosevelt Hospital Center, New York

Jean-Michel Guerin, M.D.—Groupe de Recherche sur les Maladies Immunitaires en Haiti, Port-au-Prince

Harry W. Haverkos, M.D.—AIDS Activity, Centers for Disease Control, Atlanta

N. Patrick Hennessey, M.D.—Dermatologist, private practice, New York

George Hensley, M.D.—Director, Autopsy Services, Department of Pathology, University of Miami School of Medicine, Miami

Leon W. Hoyer, M.D.—Chief, Hematology Division, University of Connecticut Health Center, Farmington, Connecticut

Harold Jaffe, M.D.—Chief, Epidemiology Section, AIDS Activity, Centers for Disease Control, Atlanta

Joyce Johnson, D.O.—AIDS Activity, Centers for Disease Control, Atlanta

Dennis Juranek, D.V.M.—Director, Parasitology Division, Centers for Disease Control, Atlanta

Simon Karpatkin, M.D.—Professor of Medicine, New York University Medical Center, New York

Hal Kooden, Ph.D.—psychologist, New York

Waclaw Kornaszewski, M.D.—Professor of Medicine, National University Hospital, Kinshasa, Zaire

Larry Kramer—novelist, Cofounder of Gay Men's Health Crisis, New York

Sheldon Landesman, M.D.—Assistant Professor of Medicine, Division of Infectious Diseases, Downstate Medical Center, State University of New York, New York

Michael Lange, M.D.—St. Luke's–Roosevelt Hospital Center, New York

Linda Laubenstein, M.D.—Assistant Professor of Clinical Medicine, New York University School of Medicine, New York

Arthur S. Levine, M.D.—Scientific Director, National Institute of Child Health and Human Development, Bethesda, Maryland

Joe Lusi, M.D.—Chef du Zone, Eastern Region, Zaire

Pearl Ma, Ph.D.—Chief of Microbiology, St. Vincent's Hospital, New York

Clyde McAuley, M.D.—Medical Director, Alpha Therapeutic Corporation, Los Angeles

Adrian Marcel, M.D.—private practice, New York

Michael Marmor, Ph.D.—Research Associate Professor, Department of Environmental Medicine, New York University School of Medicine, New York

Lawrence Mass, M.D.—Medical Director, Greenwich House West, New York

Usha Mathur, M.D.—Attending Physician, Infectious Diseases, Beth Israel Medical Center, New York

Jay E. Menitove, M.D.—Medical Director, Southwestern Wisconsin Blood Center, Milwaukee

Craig Metroka, M.D.—Clinic Fellow, New York Hospital–Cornell Medical Center, New York

Luc Montagnier, M.D.—Head, Viral Oncology Unit, Pasteur Institute, Paris

Lee Moskowitz, M.D.—Cedars Medical Center, Miami

James Oleske, M.D.—Director of Immunology, St. Michael's Medical Center, Newark, New Jersey

Roland Perry, D.Sc., M.D.—Associate Professor of Medicine, St. Vincent's Hospital, Darlinghurst, Australia

Larry Puchall, Ph.D.—psychologist, Washington, D.C.

Gerald Quinnan, M.D.—Director, National Center for Drugs and Biologics, Federal Drug Administration, Bethesda, Maryland

Oscar D. Ratnoff, M.D.—Professor of Hematology, Case Western Reserve University School of Medicine, Cleveland

Robert Redfield, M.D.—Walter Reed Hospital, Washington, D.C.

Mel Rosen—Director, Gay Men's Health Center, New York

Arye Rubinstein, M.D.—Director, Albert Einstein AIDS Research Program, Albert Einstein College of Medicine, New York

Caitlin Ryan, M.S.W.—Director of Patient Services, Whitman-Walker Clinic, Washington, D.C.

Albert Sabin, M.D.—private practice, Albuquerque, New Mexico

Bijan Safai, M.D.—Chief, Dermatology Service, Memorial Sloan-Kettering Cancer Center, New York

Yves Savain—Head, Haitian Task Force, Miami

Helen Scheitinger—Director, Homes for AIDS Patients, Shanti Project, San Francisco

Gene Shearer, M.D.—Immunology Branch, National Cancer Institute, Bethesda, Maryland

Susan Steinmetz—Staff Member, Subcommittee on Intergovernmental Relations, U.S. Congress, Washington, D.C.

Cladd Stevens, M.D.—Laboratory of Epidemiology, New York Blood Center, New York

Guy de Thé, M.D.—Université Claude Bernard, Centre National de la Recherche Scientifique, Paris

Jan Vilcek, M.D.—Professor of Microbiology, New York University School of Medicine, New York

Bruce Voeller, Ph.D.—Founder, National Gay Task Force, Washington, D.C.

Paul A. Volboerding, M.D.—Codirector, KS Clinic, University of California, San Francisco

Joyce Wallace, M.D.—Attending Physician, St. Vincent's Hospital, New York

Joel Weisman, D.O.—Internal Medicine, private practice, Los Angeles

Tim Westmoreland—Legal counsel to Congressman Henry Waxman, Washington, D.C.

Mark Whiteside, M.D.—Institute of Tropical Medicine, Miami

Daniel William, M.D.—Internal Medicine, private practice, New York

Michael Wilson—Coordinator, Public Health Education, M.D. Anderson Hospital and Tumor Institute, Houston

Susan Zolla-Pazner, Ph.D.—Chief, Clinical Immunology, Manhattan V.A. Hospital, New York

Resource Directory

For the most current and complete listings of AIDS-related organizations and hotlines, contact either the Computerized AIDS Information Network, 1213 N. Highland Avenue, Hollywood, CA 90038, (213) 464-7400, ext. 277, or the National Gay Task Force, 80 Fifth Avenue, Suite 1601, New York, NY 10011, (800) 221-7044 or (212) 807-6016.

AIDS-RELATED ORGANIZATIONS AND HOTLINES

BY STATE (U.S.)

Arizona

Phoenix:
Phoenix Hotline, (602) 957–0363

Tucson:
Tucson Alternative Lifestyle Health Association, P.O. Box 2883, 85702-2883, (602) 573-0096
Tucson Gay Health Project, P.O. Box 2807, 85720
Tucson Gay Men's Clinic, 101 W. Irvington Rd., 85714

California

Berkeley:
Gay Men's Health Collective, 2339 Durant Ave., 94704-1670, (415) 644-0425

Pacific Center for Human Growth, 2712 Telegraph Ave., 94705, (415) 841-6224/548-8283

Garden Grove:

AIDS Response Program, Gay & Lesbian Community Services Center of Orange County, 12832 Garden Grove Blvd., Suite 200, 92643, (714) 534-0862; Hotline: (714) 534-3261

Long Beach:

Long Beach AIDS Service Group, 2025 E. 10th St., 90804, (213) 439-3948

Long Beach Department of Health, 2655 Pine Ave., 90806, (213) 427-7421, ext. 274

Los Angeles:

Aid for AIDS, 7985 Santa Monica Blvd., Suite 109-171, West Hollywood, 90046, (213) 461-6959

AIDS Project/Los Angeles, 937 N. Cole, #3, 90038, (213) 871-1284; Hotlines: (213) 871-AIDS, and (800) 922-AIDS (Toll-free for S. California only)

Gay and Lesbian Community Services Center, 1213 N. Highland Ave., Hollywood, CA 90038, (213) 464-7276, ext. 267

People with AIDS—Los Angeles, c/o Trainor, 1752 North Fuller, 90046

Shanti Foundation, (213) 874-2030

South CA Mobilization Against AIDS, 1428 N. McCadden Pl., 90028, (213) 463-3928

Sacramento:

Sacramento AIDS/KS Foundation, 900 K St., #103, 98514, (916) 488-AIDS

San Diego:

Owen Clinic, University of CA Medical Center, 255 Dickinson St., 92103, (619) 294-3995

San Diego AIDS Project, P.O. Box 81082, 92138, (619) 294-AIDS; Hotline: (619) 260-1304

Beach Area Community Clinic, 3705 Mission Blvd., 92109, (619) 488-0644

San Francisco:

AIDS InterFaith Network, 890 Hayes St., 94117, (415) 558-9644

AIDS Worried Well Group, Operation Concern, 1853 Market St., 94103

Lesbian & Gay Health Services Coordinating Committee, Department of Public Health, 101 Grove, 94102, (415) 558-2541

People with AIDS/SF, 1040 Ashbury #5, 94117, (415) 665-3787

San Francisco AIDS Foundation, 333 Valencia St., 4th floor, 94103-0960, (415) 864-4376; Hotline: (415) 863-2437

Shanti Project, 890 Hayes St., 94117, (415) 558-9644

San Jose:

AIDS Foundation of Santa Clara County, 715 N. First St., Suite 10, 95112, (408) 298-AIDS

San Luis Obispo

San Luis Obispo AIDS Task Force, 2180 Johnson Ave., 93401, (805) 549-5540

Quadri-Counties: (For Santa Barbara, San Luis Obispo, Ventura, and Kern Counties)

Quadri-County AIDS Task Force, 300 San Antonio Rd., Santa Barbara, 93110, (805) 967-2311, ext. 455

Colorado

Denver:

Colorado AIDS Project, Gay & Lesbian Community Center of CO, 1615 Ogden St., 80218, (303) 837-0166

Gay & Lesbian Health Alliance of Denver, P.O. Box 6101, 80206

Connecticut

Hartford:

Hartford Gay Health Collective, 281 Collins St., 06105, (203) 724-5194

AIDS Coordinator, State Department of Health Services, 150 Washington St., 06106, (203) 566-5058

New Haven:

AIDS Project/New Haven, P.O. Box 636, 06503, (203) 624-2437

Delaware

Wilmington:
Gay & Lesbian Alliance of Delaware, P.O. Box 9218, 19809, (302)
764-2208

District of Columbia

AIDS Education Fund, Whitman-Walker Clinic, 2335 18th St., N.W.,
Washington, D.C. 20009, (202) 332-5295
D.C. AIDS Task Force, (202) 833-3234

Florida

Key West:
AIDS Action Committee, Florida Keys Memorial Hospital, P.O.
Box 4073, 33041

Miami:
Health Crisis Network, (305) 358-4357

Tampa:
Tampa Bay AIDS, P.O. Box 350217, 33695-0217

Ft. Lauderdale:
Health Crisis Network, (305) 674-7530

Georgia

Atlanta:
AID Atlanta, 1132 West Peachtree St., N.W., Suite 112, 30309,
(404) 872-0600; Hotline: (404) 892-2459
People With AIDS—Atlanta, c/o G. McGahee, 1235 Monroe Dr.
#1, 30306

Illinois

Chicago:
AIDS Action Project, Howard Brown Memorial Clinic, 2676 N.
Halsted, 60614, (312) 871-5777
People with AIDS—Chicago, c/o Hall, 3414 N. Halstead St., 60657
Sable/Sherer Clinic, Fantus Health Center of Cook County Hos-
pital, 1835 W. Harrison, 60612, (312) 633-7810

Kentucky

Lexington:
Lexington Gay Services Organization, P.O. Box 11471, 40511, (606) 231-0335

Louisiana

New Orleans:
Crescent City Coalition, Louisiana Community Center, 1022 Barracks St., 60116, (504) 244-6900
Health Department, (504) 525-1251

Maryland

Baltimore:
Baltimore Health Education Resource Organization, Medical Arts Building/Read & Cathedral Sts., 21201, (301) 947-2437
Gay Community Center of Baltimore Health Clinic, 241 W. Chase St., 3rd floor, 21201, (301) 837-2050

Massachusetts

Boston:
AIDS Action Project, Fenway Community Health Center, 16 Haviland St., 02115, (617) 267-7573
Mayor's Committee on AIDS, City Hall, 02201, (617) 424-5916

Dorchester:
Haitian Committee on AIDS in Massachusetts, 117 Harvard St., 02124

Michigan

Detroit:
Palmer Clinic, 22750 Woodward, 48220

Royal Oak:
Wellness Networks, Inc., P.O. Box 1046, 48068, (800) 521-7946, ext. 3582; in Michigan: (800) 482-2404, ext. 3582

Minnesota

Minneapolis:
Minnesota AIDS Project, 1010 Park Avenue, 55408, (612) 371-0180

Missouri

St. Louis:
AIDS Task Force, c/o Dept. of Anthropology, Washington University, 63130

Nevada

Las Vegas:
Southern Nevada Social Services, P.O. Box 71014, 89109, (702) 733-9990

New Jersey

Newark:
St. Michael's Hospital, (201) 596-0767

New Brunswick:
New Jersey Lesbian & Gay AIDS Awareness, (201) 877-5525

Trenton:
New Jersey Department of Health, Division of Communicable Diseases, AIDS Office, Health & Agriculture Building, 08625, (609) 292-7300

New Mexico

Albuquerque:
AIDS Task Force Hotline, (505) 827-3201
Common Bond, P.O. Box 1191, 87131, (505) 266-8041

Espanola:
New Mexico Physicians for Human Rights, P.O. Box 1361, 87532, (505) 753-2779

Santa Fe:
AIDS Task Force, P.O. Box 968, 87504; Hotline: (505) 827-3201
STD Clinic, 605 Letrado, (505) 827-9660

New York
Statewide Hotline: (800) 462-1884

Albany:
AIDS Council of Northeastern New York, (518) 445-2437

Brooklyn:
Haitian Coalition of AIDS, 255 Eastern Pkwy., Brooklyn 11238, (718) 735-3568; Hotline: (718) 855-0972

Buffalo:
Western New York AIDS Program, P.O. Box 38, Bidwell Stn., 14222, (716) 881-1275; Hotline: (716) 881-2347

New York City:
AIDS Resource Center, 235 W. 18th St., 10011, (212) 206-1414

Gay Men's Health Crisis, Box 274, 132 W. 24th St., 10011, (212) 807-6655; Hotline: (212) 807-6655

New York AIDS Action, 263A W. 19th St., Room 125, 10011, (212) 242-3900

New York AIDS Network, 125 Barrow St., 10014, (212) 206-1003

Office of Gay & Lesbian Health, NYC Department of Health, 125 Worth St., Room 604, 10013, (212) 566-6110 or 285-9503

People with AIDS—NY, Box G27, 444 Hudson St., 10014, (212) 242-0545

Wipe Out AIDS, 227 Waverly Pl., 10014, (212) 675-1412

Rochester:
AIDS Rochester, 153 Liberty Pole Way, 14604, (716) 232-7181; Hotline: (716) 244-8640

South Hampton:
East End Gay Organization for Human Rights, P.O. Box 87, 11968

Stony Brook:
Long Island AIDS Project, School of Allied Health Professions, Health Sciences Center, SUNY, 11794, (516) 444-AIDS

White Plains:
Mid-Hudson AIDS Task Force, Gay Men's Alliance, 255 Grove St., 10601

North Carolina

Durham:
AIDS Project, Lesbian & Gay Health Project, P.O. Box 11013, 27703, (919) 286-0079

Wilmington:
GROW, A Community Service Corporation, P.O. Box 4535, 28406, (919) 675-9222

Ohio
Statewide Hotline: (800) 322-2437

Cincinnati:
Ambrose Clement Health Clinic, 3101 Burnet Ave., 45229, (513) 352-3143
AIDS Task Force, (513) 352-3138

Cleveland:
Cleveland AIDS Foundation, 11900 Edgewater Dr., #907, Lakewood, 44107

Columbus:
Open Door Clinic, 237 E. 17th St., 43201, (614) 294-6337

Oklahoma

Oklahoma City:
Health Guard Foundation, 2135 N.W. 39th St., 73112, (405) 525-9333
Oklahoma for Human Rights, 4107 E. 2nd Pl., 74112

Oregon

Portland:
Cascade AIDS Project, Phoenix Rising Foundation, 408 S.W. 2nd, Room 407, 97204, (503) 223-8299
AIDS Task Force, 105 35 N.E. Glisan, 97220, (503) 254-8812

Pennsylvania

Philadelphia:
Philadelphia AIDS Task Force, P.O. Box 7259, 19101, (215) 232-8055

Texas

Dallas:

AIDS Project, (214) 351-4335

The Holloway Foundation, 13777 N. Central Expressway, Suite 401, 75243, (214) 987-9023

Oak Lawn Counseling Center AIDS Project, 3409 Oak Lawn, Suite 202, 75219, (214) 528-2081

People with AIDS—Dallas, c/o Oak Lawn Counseling Center, Attn: P. Gerber, 3409 Oak Lawn, Suite 202, 75219

Houston:

Committee for Public Health Awareness, P.O. Box 3045, 77253, (713) 528-6333

KS/AIDS Foundation of Houston, 1001 Westheimer, Suite 193, 77006, (713) 524-AIDS

Montrose Clinic, 803 Hawthorne, 77006, (713) 227-6505

Utah

Statewide Hotline: (801) 533-0927

Washington

Seattle:

Seattle AIDS Action Project, 113 Summit Ave. E., #204, 98102, (206) 323-1229

Seattle Gay Clinic, P.O. Box 20066, 98102

Seattle-King County Department of Public Health AIDS Assessment Clinic, 1406 Public Safety Building, 610 Third Ave., 98104, (206) 587-4999

INTERNATIONAL

Canada

AIDS Committee of Toronto, c/o Hassle Free Clinic, 556 Church St., 2nd Floor, Toronto, Ontario M4Y 2E3

AIDS Vancouver, c/o 19th Floor, 355 Burrard St., Vancouver, British Columbia V6C 2J3

Centretown Community Resources, 100 Argyle Ave., Ottawa, Ontario K2P 1B6

Collective D'Intervention Communautaire Auprès des Gais, C.P. 29 Succursale Victoria, Montreal, Quebec, (514) 484-2602

Comité SIDA du Québec, 3757 rue Prud'homme, Montreal, Quebec H4A 3H8

Gay Social Service Project, 5 rue Weredale Park, Montreal, Quebec H3Z 1Y5

Gays of/Gais de Ottawa, Box 2919 Stn. D, Ottawa, Ontario M5W 1X7

England

Capitol Gay, 38 Mount Pleasant, London, MC1XOAP

France

Association des Gais Médecins, 45 rue Sedaine, 75011 Paris

The Netherlands

AIDS Policy Coordinator, Jan K. van Wijngaarden, M.D., Buro G.V.O., Prins Hendrikiaan 12, 1075 BB Amsterdam

COC—Joop van der Linden, Rozenstraat 8, 1016 NX Amsterdam

Puerto Rico

Rio Piedras:

Latin American STD Center, Centro Medico, 00922, (809) 754–8118

National Aids-Related Organizations

American Association of Physicians for Human Rights, 1050 W. Pacific Coast Hwy., Harbor City, CA 90710, (213) 548-0491

American Psychological Association, 1200 17th St., N.W., Washington, D.C. 20036, (202) 955-7600. Contact: Dr. Arnold Kahn

Association of Lesbian & Gay Psychologists, American Psychological Association, 1200 17th St., N.W., Washington, D.C. 20036, (202) 955-7600. Contact: Walter Batchelor

Gay Nurses' Alliance, 608 W. 28th St., Wilmington, DE 19802, (302) 764-2208. Contact: Jim Welch

Gay Rights National Lobby/AIDS Project, P.O. Box 1892, Washington, D.C. 20012, (202) 546-1801

National AIDS Hotline (CDC), (800) 342-AIDS

National AIDS/Pre-AIDS Epidemiological Network, 2676 N. Halsted St., Chicago, IL 60614, (312) 943-6600, ext. 424, 389. Contact: David Ostrow, M.D.

National AIDS Research & Education Foundation, 54 Tenth St., San Francisco, CA 94013, (415) 626-8784

National Association for Lesbian & Gay Gerontology, 271 Lacasa Ave., San Mateo, CA 94403, (415) 349-4537. Contact: Donald Catalano

National Coalition of Gay STD Services, P.O. Box 239, Milwaukee, WI 53201-0239, (414) 277-7671. Contact: Mark Behar

National Gay Health Coalition, 206 N. 35th St., Philadelphia, PA 19143, (215) 386-5327. Contact: Walter Lear

National Gay Task Force, 80 Fifth Ave., New York, NY 10011, (212) 741-5800. Contacts: John Boring/Jeffrey Levi

National Lesbian and Gay Health Foundation, P.O. Box 65472, Washington, D.C. 20035. Contact: Caitlin Ryan

National People With AIDS Projects, c/o AID Atlanta, 1801 Piedmont Rd., Suite 208, Atlanta, GA 30324, (404) 872-0600. Contact: Glenn D. McGahee

Women's AIDS Network, 707 San Bruno Ave., San Francisco, CA 94117, (415) 821-7984. Contact: Laurie Hauer

Miscellaneous Organizations

American Cancer Society:
Los Angeles: 2975 Wilshire Blvd., Suite 200, Los Angeles, CA 90010-1110, (213) 386-6102
National: 777 Third Ave., New York, NY 10017, (212) 371-2900
Centers for Disease Control, 1600 Clinton Rd., N.E., Atlanta, Georgia 30333

Community Cancer Control, 5410 Wilshire Blvd., Suite 1008, Los Angeles, CA 90036, (213) 938-2408

Gay/Lesbian Community Centers (check your local directory as well):

Gay Community Center of Orange County, 12832 Garden Grove Blvd., Suite 200, Garden Grove, CA 92643, (714) 859-6482

Index

budget, 221
culture materials, 225–26
master registry, 66
National Institute for Occupational
Safety and Health (NIOSH)
(CDC), 61, 70
National Institute of Allergy and
Infectious Diseases (NIAID),
214, 221
National Institutes of Health (NIH),
100, 214, 253
charges of nonresponse, 218,
219
Clinical Center, Bethesda, 43, 190,
215
meeting on viruses, 94, 95–97, 99,
101
research funding for AIDS, 218
Needles, contaminated, 126–27, 141,
143, 205
Neurons, 181
New England Journal of Medicine
(NEJM), 19–20, 72, 121, 130,
175–76, 213, 225
New Republic, 116–17, 153
New Scientist (magazine), 170
New York City, 66, 69, 79, 80
AIDS cases, 17–18, 19, 32, 204,
207–208
cluster of AIDS cases, 84–88
cost of care (AIDS patients),
213
gay population, 33–34
infant AIDS cases, 148–50
New York Funeral Directors Association, 234
New York Native, The (magazine),
240, 244
New York Review of Books, The, 223,
248
New York State Department of
Health
AIDS Newsletter, 178–79
New York Times, The, 33, 120, 123–
24, 169, 170
New York University, 97

Cancer Registry, 30
case control study, 73–75, 77,
78
University Hospital, 229, 232
Nezelof's syndrome, 149
Night sweats (symptom), 140
NIH, *see* National Institutes of Health
(NIH)
NIOSH, *see* National Institute for
Occupational Safety and Health
(NIOSH) (CDC)
Nitrites, 60
see also Amyl nitrite; Butyl nitrite
Nurses, *see* Health workers

Office of Technology Assessment,
170, 219–20, 221, 223–24,
225
OI, *see* Opportunistic infections (OI)
Oklahoma City, 66
Oleske, Dr. James, 146–48, 150–53,
154–57, 158–59, 161–62, 163
Olweny, Dr. Charles, 123
Opportunistic infections (OI), 22–23,
24, 38, 40, 41, 49, 66, 76, 147,
156, 181, 184, 186, 216
CMV as, 39
in diagnosis of AIDS, 185
in Haiti, 121
in infant AIDS cases, 159, 161
protection against, 192
selective, 43
Oral-anal contact, 72
Oral thrush, 150
Organisms, 3, 5, 44
causing opportunistic infections,
22–23
do not destroy own environment,
241

Pagano, Dr. Joseph, 97
Paine, Thomas, 210
Papovavirus, 96
Parasites, 193–94
Parasitic infections, 186
Paris, 124

U.S. Air Force, 234
U.S. Department of Health and
Human Services, 170, 218, 223,
224, 253
University of California at Los An-
geles, 215
University of California at San Fran-
cisco, 215
University Hospital, Kinshasa, Zaire,
192, 206
Urmacher, Dr. Carlos, 31

Vaccines, 5, 172, 206, 221, 223, 250,
251
for hepatitis B, 138–39
against viral diseases, 93
premature announcement of
AIDS, 168, 171
Vaccination, 45
Vaginal sex, 166
Vanga, Zaire, 206
Venereal diseases, 17, 23, 71, 227
AIDS as, 178
see also Sexually transmitted dis-
eases (STDs)
Vilcek, Dr. Jan, 53
Viral agents, 5, 197
Viral diseases, 12, 93, 101
Viral infections, 22
see also Retroviral infections
Viral replication:
inhibition of, 188, 189–90, 191
Virus(es), 3, 38, 45
as cause of AIDS (theory), 2, 4,
5, 76, 77–78, 88, 93–101, 109,
128
as cause of cancer, 8
as cause of KS (theory), 38–39
maladjusted, 101
mutations of, 57–58, 197
see also Retroviruses
Visna virus, 183
Vitamin B, 205
Vitamin B$_{12}$, 25
Voeller, Dr. Bruce, 132, 133, 139
Vogle, Charles, 27

Volboerding, Dr. Paul, 35, 181, 182,
185

Waddell, Dr. Tom, 239
Wallace, Dr. Joyce, 25–26, 27, 32,
164
Ward, Ingeborg, 57
Washington, D.C., 80
Waxman, Henry, 218, 222
Weight loss (symptom), 14, 17–18,
19, 140, 141, 150, 155, 179
Weinberg, Martin S., and Alan P.
Bell:
Homosexualities, 237–38
Weisman, Dr. Joel, 13–14, 79, 83,
246, 248
Weiss, Ted, 227–28
Western blot test, 175, 176
Westmoreland, Tim, 222
White blood cells, 44, 53, 181
Whiteside, Dr. Mark, 208
WIC (women/infants/children) pro-
grams, 212
Wickramasinghe, Chandra, 196
William, Dr. Dan, 26–27, 40, 73,
87, 89, 232, 236, 248
African genesis theory, 122, 123
Wolf, Dr. Robert, 13
Women as AIDS victims, 4, 121, 123–
24, 141, 163–64, 166, 172, 178,
197, 200
in Africa, 206–207
in Haiti, 116, 164, 165
KS in, 184
see also Lesbians; Mothers of in-
fant AIDS cases
Wooden, Wayne S., and Jay Parker:
Men Behind Bars, 239
World Health Organization, 122

Yellow fever, 62

Zaire, 122, 124, 183, 203
Zambia, 203
Zolla-Pazner, Dr. Susan, 8, 37–38,
99, 219